Manual for Eye Examination and Diagnosis

Mark W. Leitman, MD
Clinical Assistant Professor
Department of Ophthalmology and Visual Sciences
Montefiore Hospital
Albert Einstein College of Medicine
Bronx, NY, USA

TENTH EDITION

WILEY Blackwell

This edition first published 2021
© 2021 John Wiley & Sons Ltd

Edition History
9e, 2017 by John Wiley & Sons, Inc.

The right of Mark W. Leitman to be identified as the author of this work has been asserted in accordance with law.

Registered Offices
John Wiley & Sons, Inc., 111 River Street, Hoboken, NJ 07030, USA
John Wiley & Sons Ltd, The Atrium, Southern Gate, Chichester, West Sussex, PO19 8SQ, UK

Editorial Office
9600 Garsington Road, Oxford, OX4 2DQ, UK

For details of our global editorial offices, customer services, and more information about Wiley products, visit us at www.wiley.com.

Wiley also publishes its books in a variety of electronic formats and by print-on-demand. Some content that appears in standard print versions of this book may not be available in other formats.

Library of Congress Cataloging-in-Publication Data

Name: Leitman, Mark W., 1946– author.
Title: Manual for eye examination and diagnosis / Mark W. Leitman.
Description: Tenth edition. | Hoboken : Wiley-Blackwell, 2020. | Includes index.
Identifiers: LCCN 2020021835 (print) | LCCN 2020021836 (ebook) | ISBN 9781119628583 (hardback) | ISBN 9781119630623 (adobe pdf) | ISBN 9781119630579 (epub)
Subjects: MESH: Eye Diseases–diagnosis | Diagnostic Techniques, Ophthalmological | Handbook
Classification: LCC RE75 (print) | LCC RE75 (ebook) | NLM WW 39 | DDC 617.7/15–dc23
LC record available at https://lccn.loc.gov/2020021835
LC ebook record available at https://lccn.loc.gov/2020021836

Cover Design: Wiley
Cover Images: (front cover) courtesy of Carl Zeiss Meditect, Inc., (back cover) JirehDesign.com and courtesy of Stuart Green

Set in 8.5/11pt Frutiger by SPi Global, Pondicherry, India

SKY101754_032321

Contents

Preface

The first edition of this book was started when I was a medical student at N.Y. Medical College 48 years ago during the allotted 2-week rotation in the eye clinic. It was published during my first year of eye residency at Albert Einstein Medical School with assistance and encouragement from my chairman, Dr Paul Henkind. At that time, all introductory books were 500 pages or more and could not be read quickly enough to understand what was going on. With this in mind, each word of this manual is shorter and more concise. On completing it, students should understand the refraction and hundreds of the most commonly encountered eye diseases, which are discussed with respect to anatomy, instrumentation, differential diagnosis, and treatment. It is highlighted with over 600 of the best images and illustrations I have collected in the past 45 years.

The book is meant to be read in its entirety in several hours and to impart to you a foundation on which to grow and enjoy this beautiful and ever-changing specialty. The popularity of previous editions has resulted in translations into Spanish, Japanese, Indonesian, Italian, Russian, Greek, Polish, Chinese, and Portuguese as well an Indian reprint.

My special appreciation goes to Johnson & Johnson, which provided a generous grant to distribute the 7th edition to 40,000 students. I donated 60,000 copies of the 8th and 9th edition and 55,700 copies of the 10th edition to medical students. Now on with the work. Many images were generously provided by Pfizer, Wills Eye Hospital, the University of Iowa, Montefiore Hospital, and many colleagues. Elliot Davidoff, who sat next to me in medical school, and who is now assistant professor at the Ohio State University, surprised me with many unsolicited contributions, as did Lance Lyons, Glaucoma Fellow at the Mayo Clinic.

This edition has been updated with 40 new images. I hope you enjoy reading it half as much as I enjoyed writing it. I have received no monetary funding from, and I have no association with, any company whose products are mentioned in this book.

I added images of diabetic retinopathy to both the front and back covers of this latest edition so that it can be shown to patients. It will remind them of why they are making so much effort in controlling blood sugar.

I would appreciate any recommendations and images that would improve the next edition. You may email me at mark.leitman@aol.com.

Mark W. Leitman

Introduction to the eye team and their instruments

The eye exam depends on many sophisticated and costly instruments, together with highly trained professionals to operate them.

Ophthalmologist—The ophthalmologist attends 4 years of college, 4 years of medical (MD) or osteopathic (DO) school, and 3 years of specialty eye residency training. They may remain general ophthalmologists, but now, more often than not, spend an additional 1–2 years subspecializing in corneal and external disease, vitreoretinal disease, cataracts, glaucoma, neuro-ophthalmology, oculoplastic surgery, pathology, pediatric (strabismus), or uveitis.

Optometrist (OD)—The optometrist completes 4 years of college and 4 years of optometry school. They perform similar tasks to the ophthalmologist, with subspecialty fellowships similar to ophthalmology, but with stress on medical, rather than surgical skills.

Opticians (ABO, American Board of Opticians)—Opticians grind the lenses and put them in frames (laboratory optician) or fit them on the patient (dispensing optician). Their training and certification is highly variable from state to state, but often includes 2 years at a community college.

Ocularists (BCO, BRDO, FASO)—Ocularists are few in number and often learn their craft by apprenticeship. They have to pass tests for certification. Their job is to fit the rarely needed sclera shell after removal of an eye (Figs 423–426).

Ophthalmic technicians—Ophthalmic technicians have varying degrees of licensure. With medical supervision, they may take medical histories; measure eye pressure; do refractions and visual field testing; take visual activities; teach contact lens fitting; and often assist in the following diagnostic tests.

Instruments

Routine diagnostic testing is done with a slit lamp (Fig. 237) for the anterior segment and the handheld ophthalmoscope (Fig. 466) for the retina exam. Office-based optical coherence tomography (OCT) (Fig. 339) uses a light scanning device to measure the layers of the eye, and optical coherence tomography angiography (OCT A) physically defines the retinal and choroidal blood vessels. These light sources reflect a beam off ocular structures at up to 100,000 scans/s and require a clear, transparent media. A red blood cell has a diameter of 7 microns and OCT scans resolve down to 2–5 microns. Fluorescein angiography shows sequential blood flow and possible leakage of retinal blood vessels (Fig. 470). Ultrasound is an alternative to OCT for measuring structures through an opaque media (Fig. 560). A specular microscope (Figs 265 and 266) analyses the number and characteristics of the inner layer of the cornea called the *endothelium*. Corneal tomography (Fig. 73) measures the thickness and diopter power of the cornea. Treatments include lasers of different wave lengths. Argon lasers (see back cover) are preferred in the treatment of retinal disorders, and Nd:YAG lasers are used to open secondary cataracts (Figs 451 and 452) that occur after cataract extractions and to perform peripheral iridotomy for narrow-angle glaucoma (Fig. 365). SLT Nd:YAG lasers (Fig. 345) are used to treat open-angle glaucoma. Excimer lasers (Figs 60–62) change the shape of the cornea in the procedure called LASIK surgery. Femtosecond lasers help in certain parts of cataract surgery (Fig. 447) and SMILE refractive surgery (Fig. 77). Finally, the phacoemulsifier (Fig. 438) liquifies a 10-mm cataract so that it can be removed through a sutureless, 3-mm incision.

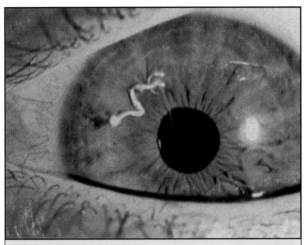

Fig 1 A seed introduced into the eye of an 8-year-old boy through a penetrating corneal wound became imbedded in the iris. Many months later, the seed became visible when it began germinating. Courtesy of Solomon Abel, MD, FRCS, DOMS, and *Arch. Ophthalmol.*, Sept. 1979, Vol. 97, p. 1651. Copyright 1979, American Medical Association. All rights reserved.

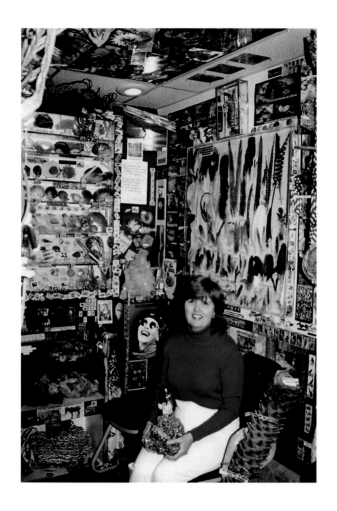

Dedicated to Andrea Kase

It is impossible to perform a good eye exam without a good support team. Andrea has enthusiastically led our team for 40 years as office manager, ophthalmic technician, and typist of all correspondence, including for the last eight editions of this book. By encouraging me to bring my collection of rocks and other exotic objects into the waiting room, she helped create a museum that my patients look forward to seeing.

Chapter 1
Medical history

History includes the patient's chief complaints
Table 1, medical illnesses, current medications,
allergies to medications, and family history of
eye disease.

Table 1 Common chief complaints	
Common chief complaints	Causes
Persistent loss of vision	**1** Focusing problems are the most common complaints. Everyone eventually needs glasses to attain perfect vision, and fitting lenses occupies half the eye care professional's day. LASIK, used to correct refractive errors, is the number one cosmetic surgery in the USA.
	2 Cataracts (Fig. 7) are cloudy lenses that commonly occur with aging. Unoperated cataracts are the leading cause of blindness worldwide. In the USA, over 3.5 million cataract extractions are performed each year. It is the number one major surgery in the USA and worldwide.
	3 Thirteen percent of American adults are treated for diabetes. Another 40% are pre-diabetic. It is the leading cause of blindness in the USA in those under 65 years of age.
	4 Age-related macular degeneration (AMD) (Fig. 516) causes loss of central vision and is the leading cause of blindness in people over age 65 (Fig 515-517 and 537). Signs are present in 25% of people over age 75, increasing to almost 100% by age 100.
	5 Glaucoma is a disease of the optic nerve that is usually due to elevated eye pressure. It mostly occurs after age 40; affects 4% of Americans over that age, with black persons affected five times as often as whites. Peripheral vision is lost first, with no symptoms until it is far advanced. This is why routine eye exams are recommended.
	6 Amblyopia affects 2–3% of children. It is due to improper use of one or both eyes in early childhood and usually resulting from eye turns (strabismus) or uncorrected refractive errors.
Transient loss of vision lasting less than ½ hour, with or without flashing lights	In younger patients, think of migrainous spasm of cerebral arteries. With aging, consider emboli from arteriosclerotic plaques. Simultaneous symptoms in both eyes often direct one to a brain etiology. Dry eye is also the common cause of on–off loss of vision.
Floaters	Almost everyone will at some time see shifting spots due to suspended particles in the normally clear vitreous. They are usually physiologic, but may result from hemorrhage, retinal detachments, or other serious conditions (Figs 556 and 557).

(Continued)

Manual for Eye Examination and Diagnosis, Tenth Edition. Mark W. Leitman.
© 2021 John Wiley & Sons Ltd. Published 2021 by John Wiley & Sons Ltd.

Table 1 (Continued)

Flashes of light (photopsia)	The retina accounts for 84% of complaints, which are usually unilateral. Simple sparks are most often due to vitreous traction on the retina (Figs 562, 568 and 570). Insults to the visual center in the brain (16%) are most often migrainous, but ministrokes, especially in the elderly, must be considered. Cerebral causes are often bilateral, with more formed images, such as zigzag lines. With aging a transient unilateral visual loss often viewed as a curtain coming down (referred to as amaurosis fugax) is most often due to a cholesterol embolus liberated from an arteriosclerotic plaque in the carotid artery (Figs 81, 143, 582 and 584-586). In older individuals transient bilateral blurring of vision is often due to decreased blood flow at the posterior circulation to the brain. A blood clot from the the heart as might occur from atrial fibrillation, a cholesterol embolus or obstruction to flow through vertebral artery in the neck should be considered. A common cause of transient blurring of vision especially in the elderly could be due to dry eye which should be considered before pursuing an extensive vascular workup. It is often associated with a gritty irritated eye relieved by artificial tears and corneal edema noted at the slit lamp (Fig. 248). Another clue to distinguish dry eye from blood flow causes is the sometimes associated neurologic symptoms such as headache, vertigo, muscle numbness or weakness or slurred speech associated with the latter etiology.
Night blindness (nyctalopia)	Nyctalopia usually indicates a need for spectacle change, but also commonly occurs with aging and cataracts. Rarer causes include retinitis pigmentosa and vitamin A deficiency.
Double vision (diplopia)	Strabismus, which affects 4% of the population, is the condition where the eyes do not look in the same direction. This binocular diplopia disappears when one eye is covered. In straight-eyed persons, diplopia is often confused with blurry vision or caused by hysteria or a beam-splitting opacity in one eye that does not disappear by covering the other eye.
Light sensitivity (photophobia) and corneal diseases (Table 9, p. 94)	Usually, a normal condition treated with tinted lenses, but could result from inflammation of the eye or brain; internal reflection of light in lightly pigmented or albinotic eyes (Figs 540–542); or dispersion of light by mucous, lens, and corneal opacities, or retinal degeneration.
Itching	Most often due to allergy, dry eye, and lid margin infections (blepharitis) (Figs 212 and 213).
Headache	Headache patients present daily to rule out eye causes and to seek direction.
	1 Headache due to blurred vision or eye-muscle imbalance worsens with the use of eyes.
	2 Tension causes 80–90% of headaches. They typically worsen with anxiety and are often associated with bilateral temple and neck pain.
	3 Migraine often occurs in families and affects in 20% of women and 10% of men. This recurrent pounding headache, often lasting for hours, but less than a day, is sometimes accompanied by nausea, bilateral blurred vision, and flashing, zigzag lights (Fig. 141). It is relieved by sleep and may be aggravated by bright light, stress, and certain foods, especially with nitrates and nitrites (Fig. 141).
	4 Sinusitis causes a dull ache about the eyes and occasional tenderness over a sinus (Fig. 223). There may be an associated nasal stuffiness and a history of allergy.
	5 Menstrual headaches are cyclical.
	6 Sharp ocular pains lasting for seconds are often referred from nerve irritations in the neck, nasal mucosa, or intracranial dura, which, like the eye, are also innervated by the trigeminal nerve (Fig. 108).
	7 Headaches that awaken the patient and are prolonged or associated with focal neurologic symptoms should be referred for neurologic study.

Table 1 (Continued)

Visual hallucinations	These most often occur in the elderly, especially in those with dementia, psychosis, or reduced sensory stimulation, as in blindness and deafness. Many medications, including cephalosporins, sulfa drugs, dopamines used to treat Parkinson's disease, vasoconstrictors, or vasodilators should be considered.
Increased tearing (epiphora)	Consider increased production due to emotion and eye irritation or decreased ability of a normally generated tear to drain into the nose. (Fig. 149)

Medical illnesses

Record all systemic diseases. Diabetes and thyroid disease are two that are most commonly associated with eye disease.

Diabetes mellitus

Diabetes may be first diagnosed when there are large changes in spectacle correction causing blurriness. It is due to the effect of blood sugar changes on the lens of the eye.

1 Diabetes is one of the common causes of III, IV, and VI cranial nerve paralysis. It is due to the closure of brainstem vessels. The resulting diplopia may be the first symptom of diabetes and often resolves by 10 weeks.
2 Retinopathy due to microvascular disease (see front and back cover) may result in macular edema. It is the primary reason for blindness before age 65. Patients with diabetes should have annual eye exams, because early treatment is critical. Retinopathy is rare in children before age 15.

Autoimmune (Graves') thyroid disease

This is a condition in which an orbitopathy may be present with hyper- but also hypo- or euthyroid disease.

1 It is the most common cause of bulging eyes, referred to as exophthalmos (proptosis). This is due to fibroblast proliferation and mucopolysaccharide infiltration of the orbit. A small white area of sclera appearing between the lid and upper cornea is diagnostic of thyroid disease 90% of the time (Fig. 1).

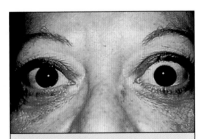

Fig 1 Thyroid exophthalmos with exposed sclera at superior limbus, due to bulging eye.

This exposed sclera may be a result of exophthalmos or thyroid lid retraction due to the stimulation of Müller's muscle that elevates the lid. Severe orbitopathy may be treated with radiation, surgical decompression of the orbit (Fig. 3), or by administering steroids orally, intravenously, or by injection into the orbit. In January 2020, the FDA approved the human monoclonal antibody, teprotumumab, to treat proptosis, strabismus, and compressive optic neuropathy from thyroid eye disease. It reduced proptosis by more than 2 mm in 71–83% of patients.

2 Infiltration of eye muscles may cause diplopia, which is confirmed by a computed tomography (CT) scan (Figs 2 and 3).

3 Exophthalmos may cause excessive exposure of the eye in the day and an inability to close the lids at night (lagophthalmos), resulting in corneal dessication.

4 Optic nerve compression is the worst complication and occurs in 4% of patients with thyroid disease. It could cause permanent loss of vision (Fig. 2) and immediate intravenous steroids should be considered when vision is threatened.

Medications (ocular side effects)

Record patient medications. Those taking the following commonly prescribed drugs are often referred to an eye doctor to monitor ocular side effects.

Hydroxychloroquine (Plaquenil), initially used to treat malaria, is now a cornerstone medication used to treat autoimmune diseases, such as rheumatoid arthritis, lupus erythematosus, and Sjögren's syndrome. It may cause retinal maculopathy with pigment changes resembling a "bull's eye" (Fig. 4). Patients should get a baseline eye exam before starting medication. It includes visual acuity, Amsler grid, color vision, and examination of the retina to rule out preexisiting maculopathy. The patient should follow up every 6 months. Depending on the dosage and the chronicity of use, the eye doctor will determine if additional tests are necessary. Risk increases

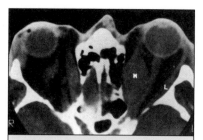

Fig 2 CT scan of thyroid orbitopathy showing fluid infiltration of the medial rectus muscle (M) and normal lateral rectus muscle (L) and proptosis. Compression of left optic nerve could cause optic neuropathy. This is called *crowded apex syndrome. Source*: Courtesy of Jack Rootman.

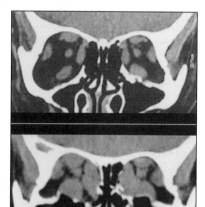

Fig 3 Orbital CT scan of Graves' orbitopathy before surgical decompression (above) and right orbital floor osteotomy (below). Often three, but rarely all four, bony walls may be opened. Note thickened extra ocular muscles. *Source*: Courtesy of Lelio Baldeschi, MD, and *Ophthalmology*, July 2007, Vol. 114, pp. 1395–1402.

if dosage exceeds 5 mg/kg. Toxicity is also related to the cumulative amount of the drug with 1% occurrence in the first 5 years and 2% after 10 years and if there is coexisting macular degeneration. These high-dose chronically treated patients may also have routine monitoring of their visual fields and optical coherence tomography (OCT) testing (Figs 463 and 464).

The retina is also adversely affected by phenothiazine tranquilizers (Fig. 5); niacin, a lipid-lowering agent and interferon, used to treat multiple sclerosis and hepatitis C (Figs 6–8).

Ethambutol, rifampin, isoniazid, and streptomycin—taken mainly for tuberculosis—may all cause optic neuropathy. The antidepressants Paxil, Prozac, and Zoloft may also cause optic neuropathy. Corticosteroids may cause posterior subcapsular cataracts (Fig. 429), glaucoma, and a reduction in immunity that may increase the incidence of herpes virus and other infections.

Flomax (tamsulosin), the most common treatment for an enlarged prostate gland, increases the complications in cataract surgery by decreasing the ability to dilate the pupil, a condition referred to as intraoperative floppy iris syndrome (IFIS). Pupillary

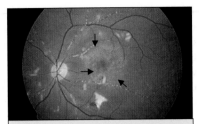

Fig 4 Bull's eye maculopathy due to hydroxychloroquine in a patient with systemic lupus. The vasculitis and white cotton-wool spots are due to lupus. *Source:* Courtesy of Russel Rand, MD, and *Arch. Ophthalmol.*, Apr. 2000, Vol. 118, pp. 588–589. Copyright 2000, American Medical Association. All rights reserved.

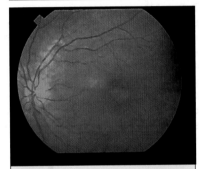

Fig 5 Phenothiazine maculopathy with pigment mottling of the macula.

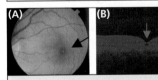

Fig 6 Tamoxifen maculopathy with crystalline deposits (A); and (B) OCT showing crystals in the fovea. *Source:* Courtesy of Joao Liporaci, MD.

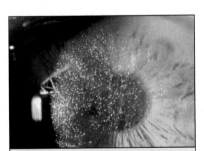

Fig 8 Besides causing maculopathy and cataracts, tamoxifen also causes crystal deposition in the cornea (keratopathy). *Source:* Courtesy of Olga Zinchuk, MD, and *Arch. Ophthalmol.*, July 2006, Vol. 124, p. 1046. Copyright 2006, American Medical Association. All rights reserved.

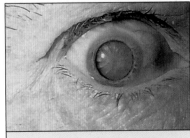

Fig 7 Tamoxifen causes cataracts.

expansion devices (Fig. 9) and additional pupillary dilating medications usually prevent complications.

Stevens–Johnson syndrome (Fig. 10) is an immunologic reaction to a foreign substance, usually drugs, and most commonly sulfonamides, barbiturates, and penicillin. Some 100 other medications have also been implicated. It often affects the skin and mucous membranes. It could be fatal in 35% of cases.

Prostaglandin analogues are the most commonly prescribed glaucoma medications. Side effects include rare, irreversible darkening of the iris (Fig. 11) and reversible reduction in orbital fat (Fig. 12) with frequent darkening and lengthening of the lashes (Fig. 13). The lash changes are often considered desirable by patients and, consequently, lead to another prostaglandin medication called *Latisse*, which is specifically prescribed for cosmetic reasons to alter the lashes.

Amiodarone (Cordarone, Pacerone), one of the most potent anti-arrhythmia drugs, and sildenafil (Viagra), tadalafil (Cialis), and vardenafil (Levitra), used to treat erectile dysfunction, have all been suspected of causing nonarteritic anterior ischemic optic neuropathy. Amiodarone almost always causes deposits in the cornea that rarely reduce vision, but may cause glare (Fig. 14).

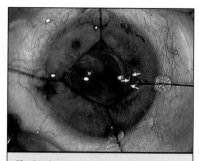

Fig 9 Iris retractors are one method used to open poorly dilated pupils during cataract surgery. Note edge of lens implant (↑) behind iris. *Source*: Courtesy of Bonnie Henderson, MD, Harvard Medical School.

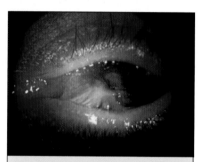

Fig 10 Stevens–Johnson syndrome with inflammation and adhesions of lid and bulbar conjunctiva. *Source*: Reprinted with permission from *Am. J. Ophthalmol.*, Aug. 2008, Vol. 1146, p. 271. Surgical strategies for fornix reconstruction. Based on *Symblepharon Severity*, Ahmad Kheirhah, Gabriella Blanco, Victoria Casas, Yasutaka Hayashida, Vadrecu K. Radu, Scheffer C.G. Tseng. Copyright 2008, Elsevier.

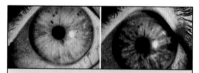

Fig 11 Irreversible darkening of a blue iris after 3 months of latanoprost (Xalatan) therapy. This is the most common drug for treating glaucoma. *Source*: Courtesy of N. Pfeiffer, MD, P. Appleton, MD, and *Arch. Ophthalmol.*, Feb. 2011, Vol. 119, p. 191. Copyright 2001, American Medical Association. All rights reserved.

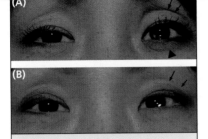

Fig 12 (A) Prostaglandin-analogue induced fat atrophy of the left orbit with sunken superior sulcus after 1 year (↑) and darkened skin (▨). Courtesy of University of Iowa, Eyerounds.org. (B) After discontinuing eye drops that had been used in the left eye for 1 year, orbital fat atrophy, darkened and lengthened lashes, and improved skin pigmentation are seen. *Source*: Courtesy of N. Pfeiffer, MD, P. Appleton, MD, and *Arch. Ophthalmol.*, Feb. 2011, Vol. 119, p. 191. Copyright 2001,

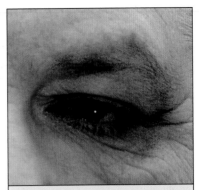

Fig 13 After long-term use of prostaglandin analogue in the left eye, the patient developed hyperpigmentation of periorbital skin, darkening and lengthening of lashes, and loss of orbital fat, causing a deepening of the upper eyelid sulcus.

Topiramate (Topamax), used to treat seizures and prevent migraine headaches, may cause angle-closure glaucoma by causing edema of the ciliary body which pushes the iris toward the cornea closing the drainage system. Immediately discontinue the drug.

Allergies to medications

Inquire about drug allergies before eye drops are placed or medications prescribed. Neomycin, a popular antibiotic eye drop, may cause conjunctivitis and reddened skin (Fig. 15).

Family history of eye disease

Cataracts, refractive errors, retinal degeneration, and strabismus—to name a few—may all be inherited. In glaucoma, family members have a 10% chance of acquiring the disease.

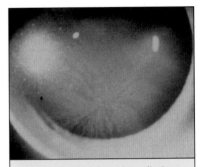

Fig 14 Epithelial deposits radiating from a central point in the inferior cornea. They occur in almost all patients with Fabry's disease, which is an X-linked systemic accumulation of a glycosphingolipid. Easily seen on a slit lamp exam, it can be the first clue in recognizing the presence of this disease, which is amenable to therapy. Indistinguishable deposits eventually appear in almost all patients using amiodarone and, less often, with hydroxychloroquine. *Source*: Courtesy of Neal A. Sher, MD, and *Arch. Ophthalmol.*, Aug. 1979, Vol. 97, pp. 671–676. Copyright 1979.

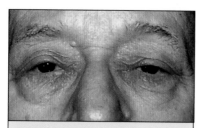

Fig 15 Neomycin allergy occurs in 5–10% of the population.

Eighty-five percent of people with migraine have an immediate relative with the disease.

A special question should be directed to a healthy lifestyle. It has been steadily worsening, causing a decrease in American lifespan to 78.6 years in 2017, compared with 82 years in Canada, Japan, and France. Fourteen percent of Americans still smoke cigarettes. It doubles the rate of cataracts, macular degeneration, and all types of uveitis. It also worsens exophthalmos due to thyroid disease, and was responsible for 480,000 deaths in America in 2018. Care must be taken in prescribing pain medications. In 2017, opioid use was the number one cause of death in America in those younger than age 50. At age 70, 80% of Americans have been diagnosed with high blood pressure. Over 50% of adults are diabetic or pre-diabetic. One-third of Americans are obese and another one-third are overweight, contributing to cancer, hypertension, and diabetes. Patients should be reminded about minimizing the consumption of red and preserved meats, salt, sugar, and saturated fats. Recommend instead an antioxidant diet rich in fruits, vegetables, beans, nuts, fish, and whole-grain cereals. Staying thin, minimizing stress, and following a routine daily exercise program should also be advocated, since even sitting at your job has been shown to shorten life span by 2 years. Mental disorders must be properly addressed since suicide, drug addiction, and alcoholism contribute significantly to morbidity. Remind patients that they must be proactive in taking responsibility for their health, and that they must become less dependent on pharmaceutical answers.

Chapter 2
Measurement of vision and refraction

It is estimated that 80% of one's sensory input is visual.

Visual acuity

A patient should read the Snellen chart (Fig. 16) from 20 ft (6 m) with the left eye occluded first. Take the vision in each eye without and then with spectacles.

Vision is expressed in a fraction-like form. The top number (numerator; usually 20) is the distance in feet at which the patient reads the chart. The bottom number (denominator) is the size of the object seen at that distance. Whenever acuity is less than 20/20, determine the cause for the decreased vision. The most common cause is a refractive error; i.e., the need for lens correction.

If visual acuity is less than 20/20, the patient may be examined with a pinhole. Improvement of vision while looking through a pinhole indicates that spectacles will improve vision.

Use an "E" chart with a young child or an illiterate adult. Ask the patient which way the ∃ is pointing. Near vision is checked with a reading card held at 14 inches (36 cm). If a refraction for new spectacles is necessary, perform it prior to other tests that may disturb the eye.

Your mission is to get them to see, while theirs is to have the vision to notice what's invisible to others.

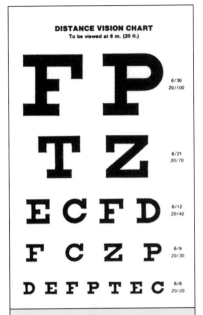

DISTANCE VISION CHART
To be viewed at 6 m. (20 ft.)

F P — 6/30 20/100

T Z — 6/21 20/70

E C F D — 6/12 20/40

F C Z P — 6/9 20/30

D E F P T E C — 6/6 20/20

Fig 16 Snellen chart measures the central eight degrees of vision.

Manual for Eye Examination and Diagnosis, Tenth Edition. Mark W. Leitman.
© 2021 John Wiley & Sons Ltd. Published 2021 by John Wiley & Sons Ltd.

Examples of visual acuity	
Measurement in feet (meters in parentheses)	*Meaning*
20/20 (6/6)	Normal. At 20 ft (6 m), patient reads a line that a normal eye sees at 20 ft.
20/30–2 (6/9–2)	Missed two letters of 20/30 line.
20/50 (6/15)	Vision required in at least one eye for driver's license in most states.
20/200 (6/60)	Legally blind. At 20 ft, patient reads line that a normal eye could see at 200 ft (60 m).
10/400 (3/120)	If patient cannot read top line at 20 ft, walk him or her to the chart. Record as the numerator the distance at which the top line first becomes clear.
CF/2 ft (counts fingers at 2 ft, 0.6 m)	If patient is unable to read top line, have the patient count fingers at maximal distance.
HM/3 ft (hand motion at 3 ft, 0.9 m)	If at 1 ft (0.3 m) patient cannot count fingers, ask if they see the direction of hand motion.
LP/Proj. (light perception with projection)	Light perception with ability to determine position of light.
NLP	No light perception: totally blind.

Record vision as follows	Key				
$\frac{V}{3}$	OD	20/70 + 1	V		Vision
	OS	LP/Proj.			Without spectacles
					With spectacles
				OD	Right eye
$\frac{V}{c}$	OD	20/20		OS	Left eye
	OS	LP/Proj.		OU	Both eyes

Optics

Emmetropia (no refractive error)

In an emmetropic eye (Fig. 17), light from a distance is focused on the retina. The cornea contributes 43.50 diopters (D) (Fig. 73) and the lens adds another 15.00 diopters but can increase by +2.50 for near focus (Fig. 377).

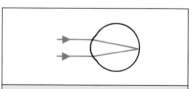

Fig 17 Emmetropic eye.

Ametropia

In this disorder, light is not focused on the retina. Three types of refractive errors, hyperopia, myopia, and astigmatism, are often inherited and occur early in life. The fourth kind called presbyopia refers to the loss ability to focus up close and typically occurs in everyone in and around the age of 43.

Hyperopia

Parallel rays of light are focused behind the retina (Fig. 18). The patient is farsighted and sees more clearly at a distance than near, but still might require glasses for viewing objects at a distance.

A convex lens is used to correct hyperopia (Fig. 19). The power of the lens needed to focus incoming light onto the retina is expressed in positive diopters (D). A positive 1 D lens converges parallel rays of light to focus at 1 m (Fig. 20).

Myopia

Parallel rays are focused in front of the retina (Fig. 21). The patient is nearsighted and sees more clearly near than at a distance. Myopia often begins in the first decade and progresses until stabilization at the end of the second or third decade. A 2016 study—the largest ever done in America—showed that in the past 50 years, the prevalence of myopia in young Americans has more than doubled to about 40%. It has been reported to be as high as 90% in Asia, where, 60 years ago, there was an incidence of 10–20%. It is strongly linked to inheritance; higher levels of education; more near work and less outdoor activity, possibly related to not enough sunlight. A concave negative lens (Fig. 23), which diverges light rays, is used to correct this condition.

Myopia may be due to increased curvature of the cornea or the human lens, but is more often due to elongation of the eye. In axial myopia, the retina is sometimes stretched so much that it pulls away from the optic disk (see Figs 472A and 472B) and may cause retinal or scleral thinning (Fig. 317) that

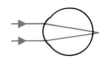

Fig 18 A hyperopic eye often has a shorter than normal axial length creating a crowded anterior segment with a smaller space between this iris and cornea. This is referred to as a narrow-angle (compare Figs 328 and 329). This may obstruct the egress of aqueous from the eye resulting in elevated eye pressure (angle-closure glaucoma. Figs 362-364). An attack may be precipitated by dilation of the pupil caused by medication or stress.

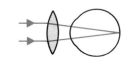

Fig 19 Hyperopic eye corrected with convex lens.

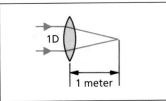

Fig 20 Parallel rays focused by 1 D lens.

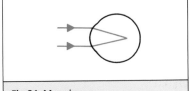

Fig 21 Myopic eye.

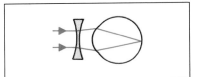

Fig 23 Myopic eye corrected by concave lens.

could result in retinal holes or detachments. This is more common in myopic eyes of –6.00 D (high myopia) and most common if greater than –10.00 D (pathologic myopia) (Fig. 22). Severe loss of vision could also be due to patches of complete atrophy of the retina or from choroidal neovascularization in 10% of those eyes (Figs 522 and 527) causing a condition similar to wet age-related macular degeneration. Glaucoma and cataract are also more common in pathologic myopia.

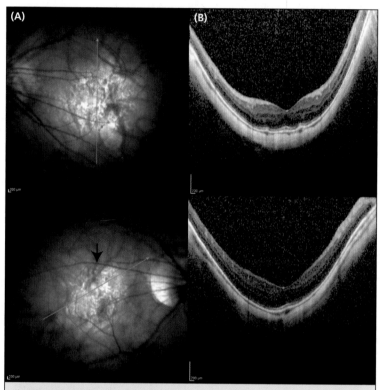

Fig 22 OCT of pathologic myopia showing: A—degeneration of macula; and B—increased axial length. The choroid may be thickened from neovascularization. Fig. 524. *Source:* Courtesy of University of Iowa, Eyerounds.org.

Astigmatism

In this condition, which affects 85% of people, the eye, rather than having a spherical shape like a basketball, is instead shaped like a football. Rays entering the eye are not refracted uniformly in all meridians. Regular astigmatism occurs when the corneal curvature is uniformly different in meridians at right angles to each other. It is corrected with spectacles. For example, take the case of astigmatism in the horizontal (180°) meridian (Fig. 24). A slit beam of vertical light (AB) is focused on the retina, and (CD) anterior to the retina. To correct this regular astigmatism, a myopic cylindrical lens (Figs 25 and 26) is used that diverges only CD.

Irregular astigmatism is caused by a distorted cornea, usually resulting from an injury or a disease called keratoconus (see Figs 43, 284, and 285).

Presbyopia

This is a decrease in near vision, which occurs in all people at about age 43. The normal eye has to adjust +2.50 D to change focus from distance to near. This is called *accommodation* (Fig. 377) and is accomplished when the shape of the lens becomes more convex. The eye's ability to accommodate decreases from +14 D at age 14 to +2 D at age 50.

Middle-aged persons are given reading glasses with plus lenses that require updating with age.

The additional plus lens in a full reading glass (Fig. 27) blurs distance vision. Half glasses (Fig. 28) and bifocals (Fig. 29) are options that allow for clear distance vision when looking up. No-line progressive bifocals are more attractive, and also allows for vision at the middle distance of 1 meter from the eye, but is more expensive.

40–45 years	+1.00	to	+1.50 D
50 years	+1.50	to	+2.00 D
Over 55 years	+2.00	to	+2.50 D

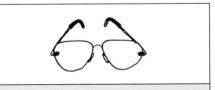

Fig 27 Full reading glass blurs distance vision.

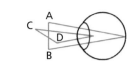

Fig 24 Myopic astigmatism. For explanation, see text.

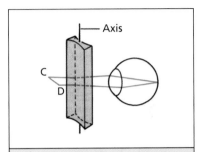

Fig 25 Myopic astigmatism corrected with a myopic cylinder, axis 90°.

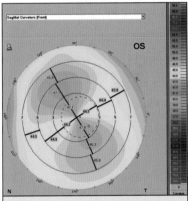

Fig 26 Tomographic image of corneal astigmatism with the steepest power +47.70 D at axis 120° and the flattest +44.51 D at 30°. To correct this myopic astigmatic error, a −3.00 D myopic cylindrical lens would be placed in the spectacle at 30°. *Source*: Courtesy of Richard Witlin, MD.

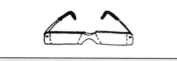

Fig 28 Half glasses.

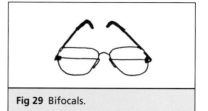

Fig 29 Bifocals.

Refraction

Refraction is the technique of determining the lenses necessary to correct the optical defects of the eye.

Trial case and lenses

The lens case (Fig. 30) contains convex and concave spherical and cylindrical lenses. The diopter power of spherical lenses and the axis of cylindrical lenses are recorded on the lens frames.

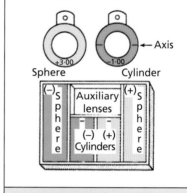

Fig 30 Lens case with red concave and black convex lenses.

Trial frame

The trial frame (Fig. 31) holds the trial lenses. Place the strongest spherical lenses in the compartment closest to the eye because the effective power of the lens varies with its distance from the eye. Place the cylindrical lenses in the compartment farthest from the eye so that the axis can be measured on the scale of the trial frame (0–180°). Some prefer using a phoropter (Fig. 32) that dials lenses in front of the patient instead of manually exchanging lenses from the lens case.

Streak retinoscopy ("flash")

This is the objective means of determining the refractive error in all patients before beginning a subjective refraction. It is the primary means to determine eyeglass prescriptions in infants and illiterate persons who cannot give adequate subjective responses. In these two instances, cyclogel 1% (Table 15, p. 147) may be instilled to prevent lens changes due to accommodation that can alter the findings.

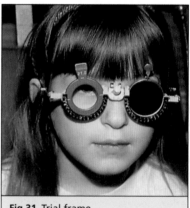

Fig 31 Trial frame.

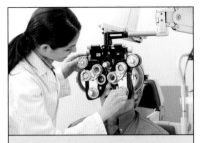

Fig 32 Phoropter dials in lenses instead of manual placement in trial frame. *Source*: Tyler Olsen/Shutterstock.com.

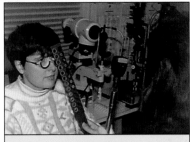

Fig 33 Streak retinoscope.

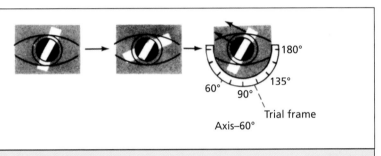

Fig 34 Retinoscopic determination of the axis of astigmatism.

Hold the retinoscope (Fig. 33) at arm's length from the eye and direct its linear beam onto the pupil. To determine the axis of astigmatism, rotate the beam until it parallels the pupillary reflex (Fig. 34), then move it back and forth at that axis, as demonstrated in Fig. 35.

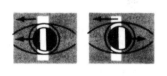

Fig 35 Pupillary reflex with motion and against motion.

If the reflex moves the same way that the retinoscope beam is moving ("with motion"), a plus (+) lens is added to the trial frame. If the reflex moves in the opposite direction ("against motion"), a negative (–) lens is needed. Absence of "with motion" or "against motion" indicates the endpoint. Add –1.50 D to the above findings to approximate the refractive error of the meridian. Rotate the beam 90° to refract the other axis. Computerized autorefractors are available to perform the same task (Fig. 36).

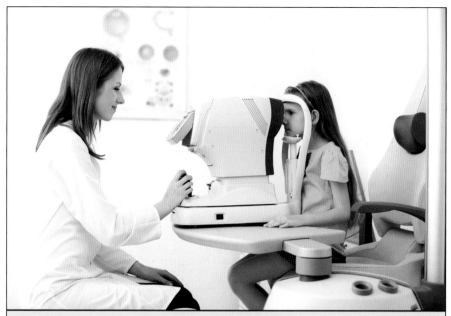

Fig 36 Computerized autorefractor may replace retinoscopy. *Source*: LovArt/Shutterstock.com.

Manifest

A manifest is the subjective trial of lenses. Place the approximate lenses, as determined by the old spectacles or retinoscopy, in a trial frame. Occlude one of the patient's eyes and refine the sphere by the addition of (+) and (–) 0.25 D lenses. Ask which lens makes the letter clearer. Next, refine the cylinder axis by rotating the lens in the direction of clearest vision. Test the cylinder power by adding (+) and (–) cylinders at that axis.

In presbyopic patients, determine the reading "add" after distance correction. The following abbreviations are used to record the results of the refraction: W, old spectacle prescription as determined in a lensometer; F, "flash," the refractive error by retinoscopy; M, manifest, the subjective correction by trial and error; Rx, final prescription, usually equal to M.

A bifocal prescription for a farsighted presbyopic patient with astigmatism is written as shown in Fig. 37. The prescription for glasses is determined by an ophthalmologist or an

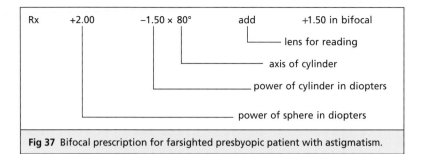

| Rx | +2.00 | −1.50 × 80° | add | +1.50 in bifocal |

- lens for reading
- axis of cylinder
- power of cylinder in diopters
- power of sphere in diopters

Fig 37 Bifocal prescription for farsighted presbyopic patient with astigmatism.

optometrist. That prescription is then given to an optician who fits it into a proper frame. They measure the interpupillary distance both near and far (Fig. 38) so that the eyes' central visual axis corresponds to the optic centers of the lens. The bifocal height for the particular frame is then determined (Fig. 39).

Plastic lenses are typically prescribed because they are lighter and have less chance of shattering. This is especially important in children. Lenses are made thicker in occupational safety glasses. Glass has the advantage of being more resistant to scratching.

For photophobia, gray tints are often prescribed because they distort all colors equally. Polaroid lenses minimize glare while driving, boating, or skiing by blocking horizontal light waves. The sun's harmful ultraviolet UVA and UVB rays may cause skin cancer (Fig. 195), photokeratitis (Fig. 248), pinguecula (Fig. 297), and pterygium (Fig. 294), while hastening the onset of cataracts and macular degeneration. Tinted lenses, including polaroid lenses, should have an ultraviolet filter added to remove 98–100% of these rays. Branded photochromic glass lenses and Transitions plastic lenses darken in sunlight and have an ultraviolet filter.

The number one ocular sports injury is from basketball. It resulted in 17,000 visits to an emergency room in a recent year. Baseball, ice hockey, and racket games are also common. Protective eye wear could prevent 90% of these sports-related injuries.

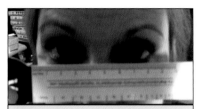

Fig 38 Measurement of interpupillary distance.

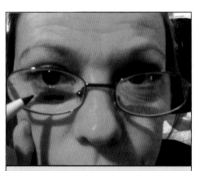

Fig 39 Determination of bifocal segment height.

Contact lenses

Plastic contact lenses, invented in 1947, are now worn by over 40 million Americans, as an alternative to spectacles, to correct myopia, hyperopia, astigmatism, and presbyopia (Figs 40 and 41).

Other uses of contact lenses include the following:

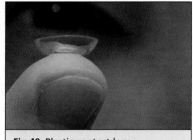

Fig 40 Plastic contact lens.

- correction of vision in cases of an irregularly shaped cornea.
- tinted lenses with or without ultraviolet protection and colored lenses for cosmetic effect (see Fig. 51).
- prosthetic artificial eyes to cover a disfigurement or enucleated socket (Fig. 426).
- bandage lenses to relieve discomfort due to blinking associated with corneal abrasions and edema.

Candidates for contact lenses

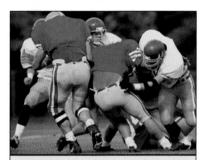

Fig 41 Contacts are beneficial for every sport.

This text will discuss soft lenses because they account for 95% of fittings. Hard and gas-permeable contacts may be preferred less often for cases of dry eye, astigmatism, and irregularly shaped corneas in keratoconus (see Figs 284 and 285).

Relative contraindications to contact lens wear:

- significant allergies,
- lid margin infections (blepharitis),
- conjunctivitis,
- dry eyes,
- very young children or elderly.

Fitting contact lenses

Keratometry

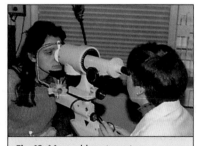

After the refraction for spectacles, the corneal curvature is measured with a manual (Figs 42 and 43) or computerized keratometer (Fig. 73). The keratometer reveals distortion of the cornea from unhealthy contact lens wear (Fig. 43) or other corneal diseases. Power

Fig 42 Manual keratometer.

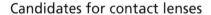

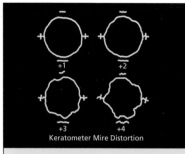

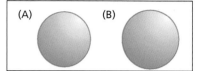

Fig 44 (A) 13.5 mm diameter. (B) 14.5 mm diameter.

Fig 43 Manual keratometer showing circular images projected on a damaged cornea with distorted keratometric readings.

(P), base curvature (BC) (Fig. 46), and diameter (DIA) (Figs 44 and 45) are the three basic variables that are usually required to order all types of soft lens (Figs 44 and 46). Curvature determines whether a flatter or steeper lens should be fitted (Fig. 57).

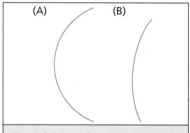

Fig 45 Contact lens properly overlapping limbus.

Determination of lens power

The power of a contact lens is not always the same as the patient's spectacle correction. Place a contact lens with the patient's spectacle power on the eye. Then, refine it with an over-refraction. The lens should completely cover the cornea and extend just beyond the entire. (corneoscleral junction; Fig. 45) and move 0.5 to 1.0 mm on each blink to distribute uniform tear film and oxygen. If adequate centration is not achieved, a different base curve or diameter may be tried.

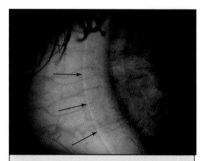

Fig 46 (A) Steep base curve, 8.2 mm. (B) Flat base curve, 9.1 mm.

Types of contact lenses

Most people wear contacts during the day only (daily wear). Sleep-in lenses (extended wear) are used less often because they have a rate of infection that is five times as great as that for daily-wear lenses. Lenses may be replaced yearly, but are more commonly disposed of every 2 weeks to 3 months ("frequent replacement") or on a daily basis ("disposable"). The frequency of replacement

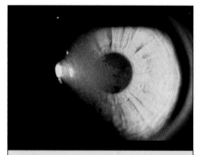

Fig 47 Mucus deposits on contact lenses.

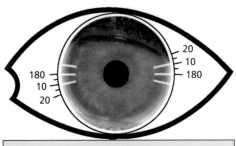

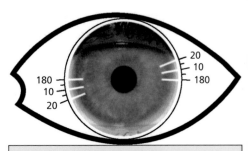

Fig 48 Lens properly aligned on eye with center marking at 180°.

Fig 49 A spectacle correction for the above eye needed an axis of 180 degrees.

depends on comfort and the rate of mucus accumulation (Fig. 47).

Astigmatism lenses (toric) are preferred when the astigmatism correction is –0.75 or more. They are elliptical in shape with markings on the 90° or 180° axis and are weighted at 6 o'clock so they do not rotate (Figs 48 and 49). When placed on the eye, these lines should align close to the 90° axis or a compensatory adjustment needs to be made in the pre-scribed lens.

But, when this contact lens, with an axis of 180 degrees, settled onto the eye, it rotated 10 degrees counterclockwise. To compensate for this unexpected rotation, a new contact lens should be placed with the axis rotated 10 degrees clockwise.

Presbyopic bifocal contact lenses are not highly successful, but may be tried for moti-vated patients—often over age 40—who have problems focusing up close (Fig. 50). An alternative to a bifocal contact lens in correct-ing a presbyopic patient is to use a standard spherical contact lens, making one eye focused for near and the other focused for distance. This is called monovision. Usually, the dominant eye with the clearest vision is chosen for distance.

The iris color can be enhanced with transpar-ent tinted soft lenses or changed to a differ-ent color with opaque tinted lenses (Fig. 51).

No patient should leave the office without feeling adept at lens insertion and removal,

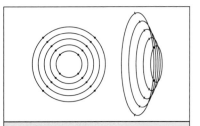

Fig 50 Bifocal contact lens with concentric zones of alternating near and far vision.

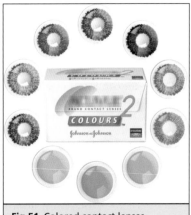

Fig 51 Colored contact lenses.

realizing the importance of good handwashing techniques, and having knowledge about the use and differences between disinfecting, cleaning, and rinsing (saline) solutions (Figs 52–54). They should also have a backup pair of glasses to be worn if eyes are irritated.

Common problems

A 2010 study of 144,799 device-associated visits of children to emergency departments showed contact lenses to be the primary cause of adverse events (23%). Corneal abrasions, conjunctivitis, and hemorrhage were most frequent.

Corneal abrasions and edema are highlighted when fluorescein dye is placed in the eye and illuminated with cobalt blue light. Areas of lost or damaged corneal epithelial cells expose the underlying stroma that takes up the dye and appears brighter (Fig. 55).

1 The upper palpebral conjunctiva is the area most often irritated by contact lenses. It is called papillary conjunctivitis (Fig. 56), and is often aggravated by contact lens deposits, especially in allergic individuals. It responds well to more frequent lens replacement.
2 The bulbar conjunctiva surrounding the cornea reddens when the cornea is being compromised, as with tight-fitting lenses (Fig. 57).
3 Infected corneal ulcers (Figs 261–263) are the most serious complication and most threatening to vision.

Orthokeratology (ortho-K) is a technique in which the refractive error is corrected by overnight sleeping with a gas permeable contact lens which flattens the cornea. It has not gained widespread popularity due to complications including infectious keratitis which is the most serious.

Refractive surgery

The refractive power of the eye may be altered by surgically reshaping the cornea (Fig. 58). Radial keratotomy, invented in the Soviet Union, began in 1978 and was the most

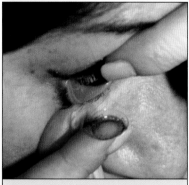

Fig 52 Place contact lens directly on the cornea using the tip of the index finger for the contact lens, the middle finger to hold the lower lid down, and the finger of the other hand to lift the upper lid.

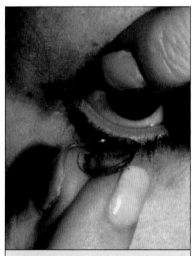

Fig 53 Remove lens by sliding it off cornea onto sclera and then gently pinching it off using thumb and index finger.

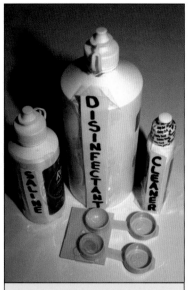

Fig 54 Contact lens solutions.

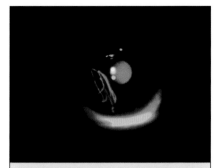

Fig 55 Fluorescein staining of the cornea.

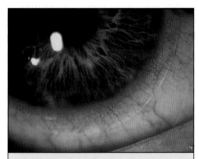

Fig 57 Limbal injection from a tightfitting lens.

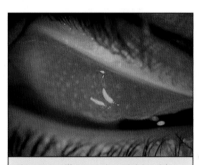

Fig 56 Papillary conjunctivitis with characteristic redness and small, whitish elevations of conjunctiva.

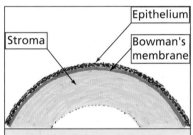

Epithelium

Stroma

Bowman's membrane

Fig 58 Normal cornea. The average central thickness is 545 μm, about half the thickness of the peripheral cornea.

popular refractive surgery in the USA until 1996 (Fig. 59). It is hardly ever performed today. In this procedure, the cornea is flattened with between four and eight radial incisions through 90% of the corneal depth. It has lost popularity due to the slow healing, the inability to accurately predict the amount of correction, variable vision throughout the day, glare, halos, infection, and corneal perforation with secondary cataract formation.

Three newer procedures—LASIK, PRK, and epi-LASIK—correct myopia hyperopia and astigmatism by using an *excimer* laser to remove corneal stroma, but this laser cannot penetrate the surface epithelium. The most popular technique to deal with this problem is called LASIK (laser in situ keratomileusis) surgery.

1 LASIK is the number one cosmetic surgery in the USA. Millions have been performed since its introduction in 1990. In this technique (Figs 60–67) a flap of epithelium and Bowman's membrane are removed with a blade (Fig. 64) or with a femtosecond laser which is different than the excimer laser (Fig. 60) used to remove stroma.

A disadvantage of LASIK is the resulting decrease in ocular rigidity. This is due to the loss of ablated stromal bed and decreased effectiveness of stroma remaining in the flap since it never completely heals. To minimize the loss of effective stroma, the goal has been to make the thinnest possible flap. Eyes with over 8 D of myopia require a lot of stromal ablation. This thinning becomes excessive and could weaken the wall of the eye resulting in ectasia (bulging) of the cornea. The average corneal thickness is 545 μm (Fig. 73) Ectasia occurs most often with pre-op corneas thinner than 521 μm and a post-op stromal bed of less than 256 μm.

LASIK damages corneal nerve fibers, which results in the commonly occurring dry eye. Another flap complication is that corneal epithelial cells can grow under the flap and may have to be removed (Fig. 67). This occurs in about 1% of primary surgeries, but in up to 23% of cases when the flap has to be lifted for a second LASIK procedure. The flap adheres poorly and can be lifted up to 20 years after its creation. The risk of complications from lifting the original flap for retreatment incrementally increases after 1 year. Trauma may dislocate this flap for many years after its creation (Fig. 66).

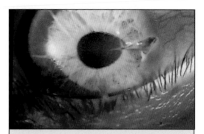

Fig 59 Rare instance of traumatic rupture of radial keratotomy wound. *Source*: Courtesy of Leo Bores.

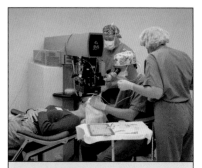

Fig 60 Excimer laser used to remove a layer of central corneal stroma.

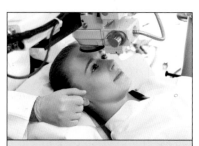

Fig 61 LASIK performed with topical anesthetic. *Source*: LovArt/Shutterstock.com.

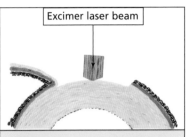

Excimer laser beam

Fig 62 LASIK: a 110 μm flap of epithelium, Bowman's membrane, and stroma is created with a blade or laser. Then, an excimer laser ablates the stroma. The post-LASIK stromal bed should be at least 250 μm to prevent excessive thinning (ectasia) prone to cause distorted vision.

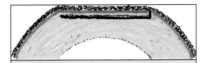

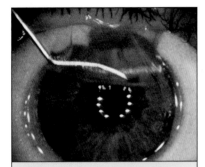

Fig 63 Sculpted cornea after LASIK with remaining Bowman's membrane.

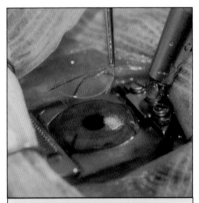

Fig 64 Superficial corneal flap created with a microkeratome. Laser creation of flap is reported to be superior. *Source*: Courtesy of Chris Barry, M.Med.Sci., and *J. Ophthalmic Photogr.*, 1999, Vol. 22, No. 1A.

Fig 65 LASIK surgery showing flap being lifted with spatula and laser beam on central cornea ablating stroma.

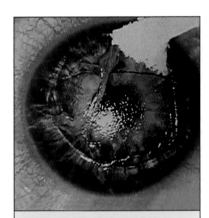

Fig 66 Late dislocation of a LASIK flap by self-inflicted injury. *Source*: Courtesy of C.K. Patel, BSC, FRC Ophth., and *Arch. Ophthalmol.*, Mar. 2001, Vol. 119, p. 447. Copyright 2001, American Medical Association. All rights reserved.

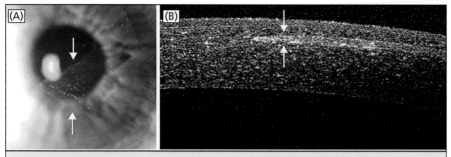

Fig 67 (A) Gray area (arrows) where epithelial cells grew under the flap. (B) OCT scan showing cells. If cells are near the central cornea, or if there is overlying melting in the peripheral cornea, the flap must be lifted and cells removed. However, the main reason for lifting the flap is to remove folds (stria). *Source*: Courtesy of V. Charistopoulos, MD, and *Arch. Ophthalmol.*, Aug. 2007, Vol. 125, pp. 1027–1036.

2 An alternative to LASIK is photorefractive keratectomy (PRK) (Figs 68–70). It eliminates the need for a flap by mechanically creating a central corneal abrasion to remove the epithelium (Figs 68 and 69). The advantage is it leaves more functioning stroma, which makes it especially useful in high myopia needing significant thinning of the cornea.

The disadvantage of PRK is pain from the abrasion that lasts about 48 hours; slower return of vision; and occasional recurrent haze. The latter may be minimized by using the topical antimetabolite mitomycin C drops during surgery which prevents cell growth.

3 The newest technique, called epi-LASIK (Fig. 71) creates an epithelial flap that includes no stroma. As a consequence, there will be more stroma remaining to contribute to ocular rigidity. However, the epithelial flap heals more slowly than the LASIK flap so that vision takes longer to recover.

All three laser techniques usually yield good results, but may be complicated most often by dry eye, but also infection, glare, halos, dry eye, over- or under-correction of refractive error, and unknown long-term effects. LASIK has been by far the most popular corneal refractive surgery for the past two decades with about 1 million procedures per year making it the most common cosmetic procedure in

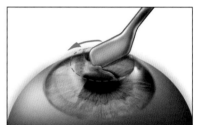

Fig 68 Removal of corneal epithelium precedes excimer laser thinning of cornea in PRK.

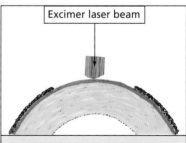

Fig 69 PRK laser ablation of Bowman's membrane and stroma after mechanical debridement of epithelium. Corneal haze sometimes could result from loss of Bowman's membrane and topical application of the anti-metabolite Mitomycin C during surgery results in clearer corneas.

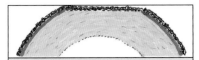

Fig 70 Sculpted cornea after PRK or epi-LASIK.

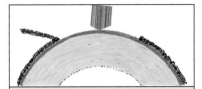

Fig 71 Epi-LASIK: creation of epithelial flap with blade followed by laser ablation of stroma.

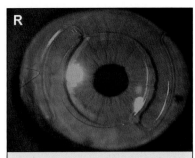

Fig 72 Phakic 6H2 anterior chamber intraocular lens to correct refractive errors. *Source:* Courtesy of Oil, Inc. surgery.

America. A recent survey revealed slightly over half of ophthalmologists would consider laser refractive surgery on themselves.

Large amounts of hyperopia (over 4 D) and myopia (over 8 D) are difficult to correct with reshaping the cornea because it becomes too thin and unstable. Intraocular lenses can be inserted inside the eye (Fig. 72) to correct these larger refractive errors, but have all the inherent risks associated with intraocular surgery.

There has to be a safe space between the implanted lens, the cornea, and the patient's natural lens or corneal edema and/or cataract could occur.

A technique called corneal limbal relaxing incisions may be used to correct astigmatism. A manual (blade) or femtosecond laser creates an accurate incision to a depth of 600 μm (80% of corneal thickness) on the steepest corneal meridian. It is usually used to correct 0.75 to 2.00 D of astigmatism (Figs 73–75). The amount of correction is determined by whether one or two incisions are used and by the depth and length of each, which may vary from 2 to 3 hours.

Small incision lenticule extraction (SMILE) is a newer alternative to LASIK for correcting −1.00 to −10.00 D of myopia and −0.75 to −3.00 D of refractive astigmatism. It is presently

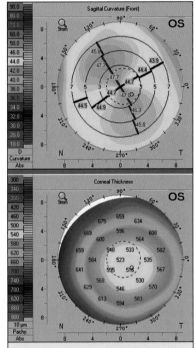

Fig 73 Tomograms of corneal topography measure 25,000 points of elevation in 5 seconds, giving the diopter power of the anterior and posterior cornea and corneal thickness. *Source:* Courtesy of Richard Witlin, MD.

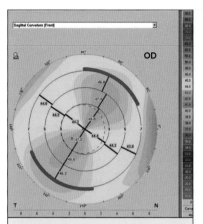

Fig 74 Limbal relaxing incision at 60° (the steepest meridian) super-imposed (in red) on a tomographic image. It corrects negative astigmatism at 150°. *Source*: Courtesy of Richard Witlin, MD.

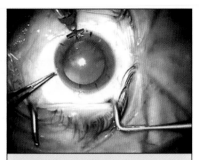

Fig 75 Manual limbal relaxing incision being created on the steepest axis at 100° to correct negative astigmatism at 10°. *Source*: Courtesy of Bonnie Henderson, Harvard Medical School.

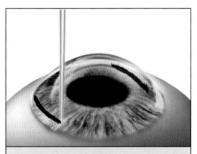

Fig 76 Femtosecond laser as an alternative to manual relaxing incision using a blade.

being evaluated for hyperopia. More than two million eyes have been treated world-wide as of 2019. A femtosecond laser (different from the excimer laser used for LASIK) is used to create a 6–7 mm corneal lenticule (Figs 77A and 77B). A dissecting spatula is then manually swept across the upper and lower borders of the lenticule to lyse any adhesions with the corneal stroma. A smooth micro-forceps is then used to remove it through a 2–4 mm tunnel incision. Collapse of the overlying corneal tissue is what causes the change in refraction. It minimizes the most troubling complications of LASIK surgery, i.e., dry eye and problems with the corneal flap. It also could be used to correct up to 10 diopters of myopia as opposed to 8 diopters with LASIK.

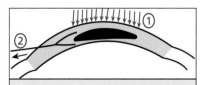

Fig 77A SMILE refractive surgery: Femtosecond laser creates a lenticule, which is removed with micro-forceps. This "pocket" surgery eliminates the need for a flap.

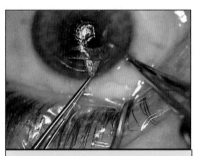

Fig 77B Removal of stromal lenticule. Be sure all remnants are removed. *Source*: Courtesy of Majid Moshirfar, MD, Moran Eye Center, Utah.

Chapter 3
Neuro-ophthalmology

The eye is part of the brain. The earliest beginnings of the brain began 550 million years ago in single-celled organisms. "Eye spots" on the cells' surface contained photoreceptor proteins that sensed light. For a description of imaging, Chapter 5. Six muscles (Table 2) move each eye around three axes. They are innervated by the III, IV, and VI cranial nerves (Table 3, Figs 78–82).

Eye movements

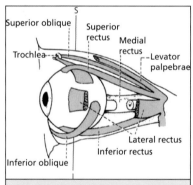

Fig 78 Lateral orbital view: adduction and abduction are around the superior–inferior axis (SI).

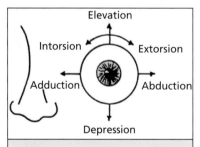

Fig 79 The eye rotates around three different axes coordinated by the action of six extraocular muscles.

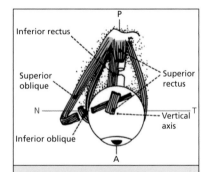

Fig 80 Superior orbital view. Elevation and depression are on the horizontal axis (NT, nasal–temporal) passing from the nasal to temporal side of the eye. Torsion is on the anterior–posterior axis (AP).

Manual for Eye Examination and Diagnosis, Tenth Edition. Mark W. Leitman.

28   © 2021 John Wiley & Sons Ltd. Published 2021 by John Wiley & Sons Ltd.

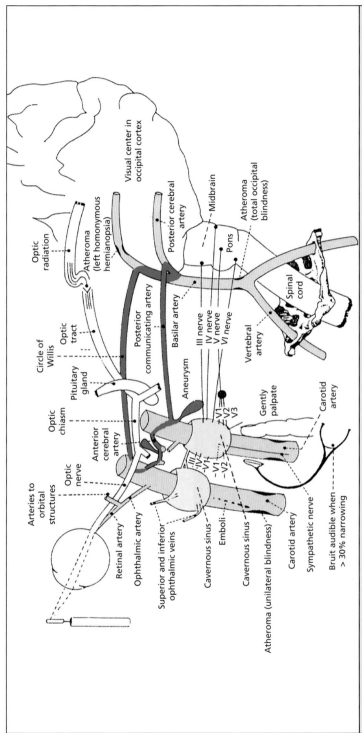

Fig 81 Blood is supplied to the brain by two vertebral arteries and two carotid arteries. The circle of Willis (green) is a cerebral arterial circle connecting the carotid to posterior cerebral arteries. It allows collateral flow if one vessel narrows. Eighty percent of ischemic strokes originate from the carotid and 20% from the vertebral or basilar circulation. The two most common cerebral aneurysms occur in this circle. The one connecting the two anterior cerebral arteries may press on the optic chiasm, sometimes causing a bitemporal hemianopsia. The other, at the junction of the carotid and posterior communicating arteries, may press on CN III, causing a dilated pupil. If the aneurysms rupture, they may cause a severe headache, a stiff painful neck, blurred or double vision, and photophobia.

Labels in figure:
- Arteries to orbital structures
- Optic nerve
- Retinal artery
- Ophthalmic artery
- Superior and inferior ophthalmic veins
- Cavernous sinus
- Emboli
- Cavernous sinus
- Atheroma (unilateral blindness)
- Carotid artery
- Sympathetic nerve
- Bruit audible when > 30% narrowing
- III, IV, V1, V2
- V1, V2, V3
- Carotid artery
- Gently palpate
- Vertebral artery
- Spinal cord
- III nerve
- IV nerve
- VI nerve
- Aneurysm
- Basilar artery
- Anterior cerebral artery
- Optic chiasm
- Pituitary gland
- Optic tract
- Circle of Willis
- Posterior communicating artery
- Optic radiation
- Atheroma (left homonymous hemianopsia)
- Visual center in occipital cortex
- Posterior cerebral artery
- Midbrain
- Pons
- Atheroma (total occipital blindness)

Table 2 Extraocular muscles.		
Muscle	*Actions*	*Neural control*
Medial rectus	Adducts	Oculomotor nerve (CN III)
Inferior rectus	Mainly depresses, also extorts adducts	Oculomotor nerve (CN III)
Superior rectus	Mainly elevates, also intorts, adducts	Oculomotor nerve (CN III)
Inferior oblique	Mainly extorts, also elevates, abducts	Oculomotor nerve (CN III)
Superior oblique	Mainly intorts, also depresses, abducts	Trochlear nerve (CN IV)
Lateral rectus	Abducts	Abducens nerve (CN VI)
Levator palpebrae	Elevates upper lid	Oculomotor nerve (CN III)
Müller's muscle	Elevates upper lid	Sympathetic nerve
Orbicularis oculi	Closes lids	Facial nerve (CN VII)

CN, cranial nerve.

Table 3 Nerves to ocular structures.		
Optic nerve, cranial nerve (CN) II	The axon of the retinal ganglion cell which transmits visual impulse from the eye to the brain	
Oculomotor nerve (CN III)	Innervates	Action
Motor (1–5)	1 Medial rectus muscle	Adducts
	2 Inferior rectus muscle	Mainly depresses, also extorts, adducts
	3 Superior rectus muscle	Mainly elevates, also intorts, adducts
	4 Inferior oblique muscle	Mainly extorts, also elevates, abducts
	5 Levator palpebrae muscle	Elevates upper lid
Parasympathetic (6 and 7)	6 Pupil constrictor muscle	Responds to light and near focus
	7 Ciliary muscle	Focuses lens for near
Trochlear nerve (CN IV)	Superior oblique muscle	Mainly intorts, also depresses, abducts
Trigeminal nerve (Fig. 108)	CN V (Fig. 108); CN V branch 1: upper lid, orbit, and nose	Sensory
	CN V branch 2: lower lid	
Abducens nerve (CN VI)	Lateral rectus muscle	Abducts

(Continued)

Table 3 (Continued)

Facial nerve (CN VII, Fig. 110)	Orbicularis muscle	Closes upper and lower lids
Sympathetic nerve (Fig. 126)	1 Müller's muscle	1 Elevates upper lid
	2 Pupil dilator muscle	2 Opens pupil in response to stress, "fight or flight," and adrenergic drugs
	3 Skin of lid	3 Sweat glands

CN, cranial nerve.

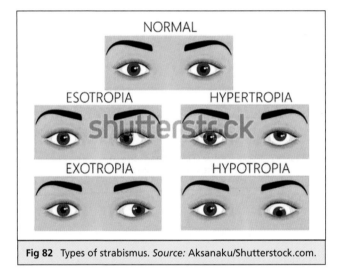

Fig 82 Types of strabismus. *Source:* Aksanaku/Shutterstock.com.

Strabismus

Strabismus (Table 4, p. 32) refers to the nonalignment of the eyes such that an object in space is not visualized simultaneously by the fovea of each eye (see Table 4).

If one eye is occluded while both eyes are fusing, the occluded eye may turn in (esophoria, noted with the letter E) or out (exophoria, X). Small phorias are usually asymptomatic. A phoria may degenerate into a tropia. A tropia is an eye-turn that occurs spontaneously. A tropia is more likely to occur as the amount of the phoria increases and as the patient's ability to compensate decreases. This occurs with tiredness later in the day and from any

Table 4 Types of eye-turn.

Esotropia (ET)	Deviation of eye nasally
Exotropia (XT)	Deviation of eye outward (temporally)
Hypertropia (HT)	Deviation of eye upward
Intermittent tropia	A phoria that spontaneously breaks to a tropia; indicate with parentheses. Example: R (ET) = right intermittent esotropia.
Constant monocular tropia	Present at all times in one eye. Example: RXT, constant right exotropia. Often associated with loss of vision, if onset is in childhood.
Alternating tropia	Either eye can deviate. Vision is usually equal in both eyes.

stimulus that dissociates the eyes, such as poor vision in one eye. Absence of a phoria (perfectly straight eyes) is termed orthophoria.

Complications of strabismus

Amblyopia

Also called lazy eye, amblyopia is decreased vision due to improper use of an eye in childhood. The two common causes are an eye-turn (strabismic amblyopia) or a refractive error (refractive amblyopia), uncorrected before age 8. In strabismus, children unconsciously suppress the deviated eye to avoid diplopia.

Strabismic amblyopia is treated by patching the good eye (Fig. 83), thereby forcing the child to use the amblyopic eye. The better eye is patched full time: 1 week for each year of age. It is repeated until there is no improvement or if the vision drops off again on cessation of patching.

Refractive amblyopia is treated by correcting the refractive error with glasses and patching the better eye. Both types must be treated in early childhood because after age 5 it is difficult to improve vision. After age 8, improvement is almost impossible, but should be tried.

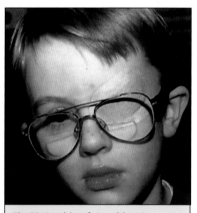

Fig 83 Patching for amblyopia.

Poor cosmetic appearance

Tropias that cannot be corrected with spectacles may be cosmetically unacceptable and the patient may desire surgery.

Loss of fusion (binocular vision)

Fusion occurs when the images from both eyes are perceived as one object, with resulting stereopsis (three-dimensional vision). Many patients with tropias never gain the ability to fuse. Finer grades of fusion are assessed by using the Wirt stereopsis test (see Fig. 84).

While wearing polarized glasses, the patient views a test card. The degree of fusion is determined by the number of pictures correctly described in three dimensions.

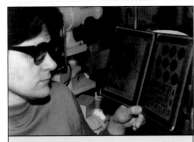

Fig 84 Wirt stereopsis.

Near point of convergence (NPC) (Fig. 85)

The NPC is the closest point at which the eyes can cross to view a near object. It is measured by having the patient make a maximal effort to fixate on a small object as it is moved toward his or her eyes. The distance at which the eyes stop converging and one turns out is recorded as the NPC. Convergence insufficiency must be considered if the NPC is greater than 8 cm. These patients may complain of diplopia or other difficulties while reading and is common in patients with Parkinson's disease. Exercises or prism glasses may help.

Accommodative esotropia (Figs 86 and 87)

When the lens of a normal eye focuses, it simultaneously causes the eyes to converge. Patients with hyperopia who are not wearing

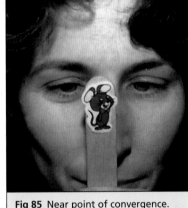

Fig 85 Near point of convergence.

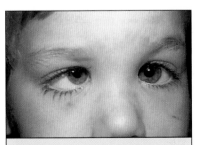

Fig 86 Accommodative esotropia.

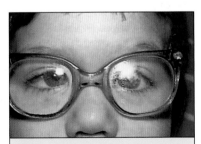

Fig 87 Accommodative esotropia corrected with hyperopic lenses.

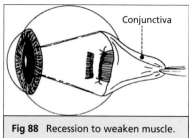

Fig 88 Recession to weaken muscle.

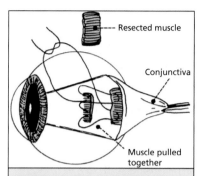

Fig 89 Resection to strengthen muscle.

glasses must focus the lens of their eye (accommodation) to see clearly near and far. This focusing stimulates the accommodative reflex, causing convergence of the eyes. When the ratio of convergence to accommodation is abnormally high, an esotropia results, which corrects with lenses.

Nonaccommodative esotropia (Figs 89 and 90)

This is due to a defect in the brain not related to the accommodative reflex. It is corrected by surgically weakening the medial rectus muscle by recessing its insertion posteriorly on the sclera or by tightening the lateral rectus muscle by resecting part of it (Figs 88 and 89). Less often, botulinum toxin is injected to weaken eye muscles. Adjustable sutures with slip knots could enable the tension on the muscle to be altered during the early postoperative period.

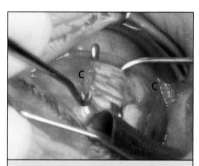

Fig 90 Strabismus surgery: after incising the conjunctiva (C), the medial rectus muscle is exposed and isolated with two muscle hooks. *Source:* Courtesy of Elliot Davidoff, MD.

An epicanthal skin fold connects the nasal upper and lower lids (Fig. 91) and is common in infants and Asians. It gives the false impression of a cross-eye, called pseudostrabismus.

Measurement of the amount of eye-turn with prisms

Ocular deviations are measured in prism diopters. When light passes through a prism, it is bent toward the base of the

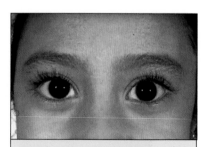

Fig 91 Epicanthal folds causing a false impression of cross-eye (pseudostrabismus).

prism. One prism diopter (1 Δ) displaces the image 1 cm at a distance of 1 m from the prism. Do not confuse prism diopters (Δ) with lens diopters (D).

In a right esotropia, the right fovea is turned temporally. To focus the light on the right fovea, a prism (apex-in) is placed in front of the right eye (Fig. 92). For an exotropia, use apex-out. *Rule:* point the prism apex in the direction of the tropia.

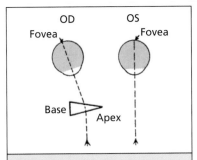

Fig 92 Right esotropia neutralized with prism (apex-in).

Prism cover test for measurement of eye-turn (Fig. 93)

The patient fixates on an object at 20 ft (6 m). When the fixating eye is occluded, the deviated eye must move to look at the target. Increasing amounts of prism are placed in front of the deviated eye until no movement is noted when the cover is moved back and forth over each eye.

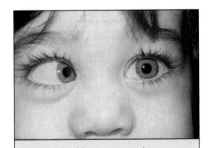

Fig 93 Prism cover test.

Hirschberg's test

When the cover test is difficult to perform on infants, the angle of strabismus can be estimated by using Hirschberg's test (Figs 94–96). As the child fixates on a point source of light, the position of the corneal light reflex is noted. Each 1 mm of deviation from the center of the cornea is equivalent to approximately 14 Δ of deviation. A reflex 2 mm temporal to the center of the cornea indicates an esotropia of approximately 28 Δ.

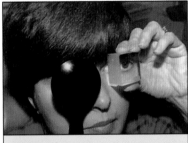

Fig 94 Hirschberg: esotropia.

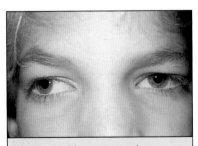

Fig 95 Hirschberg: exotropia.

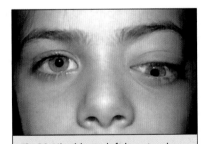

Fig 96 Hirschberg: left hypotropia.

Causes of strabismus

1 Paralytic strabismus is due to cranial nerve (III, IV, or VI) disease or eye-muscle weakness from thyroid disease, traumatic contusions, myasthenia gravis, or orbital floor fractures.
2 Nonparalytic strabismus is due to a malfunction of a center in the brain. It is often inherited and begins in childhood. Exotropias occur in over 1% of American children and may be treated for cosmetic reasons, to restore binocularity, or for headache and eye fatigue resulting from efforts to keep the eyes straight. Treatment may include eye exercises, prism glasses, or eye muscle surgery.

Demonstration of paralytic strabismus (Table 5)

In paralytic strabismus, the amount of deviation is greatest when gaze is directed in the field of action of the weakened muscle. To demonstrate underaction of any of the 12 external ocular muscles, the patient fixates on an object moved into each of the six cardinal fields of gaze (Fig. 97). Each position tests one muscle of each eye (e.g., position **3** tests the right inferior rectus and the left superior oblique muscles). In addition to observing for underaction or overaction of the muscles, ask the patient where diplopia is greatest. For exact measurements, use the prism cover test.

Most often the cause for cranial nerve (CN) III, IV, and VI paralysis cannot be confirmed, since it

Table 5 Comparison of paralytic and nonparalytic strabismus.		
	Paralytic	*Nonparalytic*
Age of onset	Usually in older persons	Usually starts before 6 years of age
Complaint since	Diplopia	Cosmetic eye-turn; less diplopia: child suppresses deviated eye
Eye-turn	Largest deviation in field of action of affected muscle	No one muscle is underactive; deviation similar in all directions
Vision	Not affected	Deviated eye may have loss of vision (amblyopia)
Plan	Neurologic workup	Ophthalmic workup

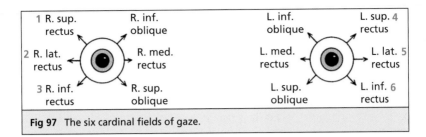

1 R. sup. rectus	R. inf. oblique	L. inf. oblique	L. sup. 4 rectus
2 R. lat. rectus	R. med. rectus	L. med. rectus	L. lat. 5 rectus
3 R. inf. rectus	R. sup. oblique	L. sup. oblique	L. inf. 6 rectus

Fig 97 The six cardinal fields of gaze.

is due to ischemia from small-vessel closure. In adults, ischemia from diabetes is the most common cause and often resolves within 10 weeks. Testing is done to rule out causes such as multiple sclerosis, aneurysms, neoplasms, and other rarer conditions, especially in younger individuals where vessel closure is not likely.

Cranial nerves III–VIII

Oculomotor nerve (CN III)

CN III paralysis (Figs 98–100) results in underaction of the inferior oblique and medial, inferior, and superior rectus muscles, resulting in an eye turned down and out. Since this nerve also innervates the levator palpebral muscle, which elevates the lid and the pupillary constrictor muscle, the lid is drooped and the pupil is dilated. CN III paralysis due to diabetes often spares the pupil.

Always examine for a dilated pupil after head trauma. CN III parallels the posterior communicating artery (see Fig. 81) so that ruptured aneurysms in the circle of Willis are a common cause of paralysis with a dilated pupil and an explosive headache (Figs 101 and 102). Also, CN III passes under the tentorial ridge in the brain and is highly susceptible to uncal herniation of the brain. Herniation may follow increased intracranial pressure from cerebral edema, hematoma, tumor, abscess, or cerebral spinal fluid obstruction. Although a dilated pupil is a more common ominous sign after head injury, small or unequal pupils could indicate serious insults to other parts of the brain.

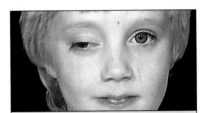

Fig 98 Right CN III paralysis. In straight gaze, eye turns down and out with dilated pupil and ptosis.

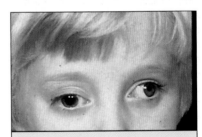

Fig 99 Inability of right eye to look to the left due to medial rectus paralysis.

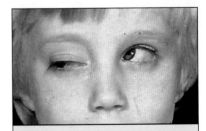

Fig 100 Inability of the right eye to look up to right due to superior rectus paralysis. *Source:* Courtesy of David Taylor.

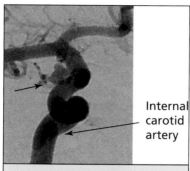

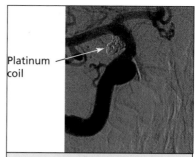
Platinum coil

Fig 101 Cerebral angiogram of right carotid artery showing a 3 mm × 4 mm posterior communicating arterial aneurysm (↑) (Figs 81 and 144). This occurred in a 50-year-old man with a subarachnoid hemorrhage and the worst headache of his life. Fifteen percent of patients with subarachnoid hemorrhages die before reaching the hospital. Aneurysms may be surgically clipped or obliterated with endovascular coiling.

Internal carotid artery

Fig 102 Stent-assisted platinum coiling embolization of aneurysm. A small electric charge is sent to the linear platinum tip when it enters the aneurysm. This charge detaches it, causes folding, and promotes thrombosis. *Source:* Courtesy of Stavropoula I. Tjoumakaris, MD, and Robert Rosenwasser, MD, Thomas Jefferson University Hospital Endovascular Neurological Surgery Department.

Trochlear nerve (CN IV)

The trochlear nerve (CN IV) innervates the superior oblique muscle. Since this muscle acts as a depressor when the eye is rotated nasally, its paralysis causes patients to have diplopia when looking down to read. Since intorsion is this muscle's main action, there is a head tilt to the opposite shoulder so that the eye doesn't have to be intorted (Fig. 103). If the doctor forces the patient's head straight (Fig. 104), the superior rectus must act as an intorter. Since the superior rectus also elevates the eye as it intorts, vertical diplopia occurs. A common cause of superior oblique muscle dysfunction is trauma since it passes through the trochlea (see Fig. 78), where it is accessible to injury due to its location just under the superior nasal orbital rim. All patients with a head tilt should be checked for trochlear nerve dysfunction.

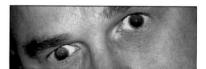

Fig 103 Left superior oblique paralysis. To avoid diplopia, head is tilted to the opposite shoulder. *Source:* Courtesy of Joseph Calhoun.

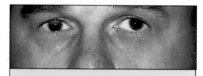

Fig 104 Paralytic left superior oblique with vertical diplopia in primary gaze. Note: sclera visible below left cornea.

Abducens nerve (CN VI)

The abducens nerve (CN VI) innervates the lateral rectus muscle that abducts the eye. Loss of function causes diplopia from the cross-eye (esotropia) greatest in its field of action (Fig. 105), less in straight ahead gaze (Fig. 106) and least or not at all in lateral gaze in the other direction Fig. 107. For this reason the patient can many times avoid diplopia by turning their head in the direction to use the normally functioning muscle or patch the abnormal eye. As this nerve may be damaged from increased intracranial pressure, one should be alert to an associated headache, nausea, and papilledema (swelling of the optic disk; see Figs 475–478.

Trigeminal nerve (CN V)

The trigeminal nerve (CN V) is the sensory nerve of the head and face (Fig. 108) and motor innervation to muscles and mastication.
V1 Ophthalmic branch: sensory to upper lid, eye, and nose.
V2 Maxillary branch: sensory to lower lid and cheek.
V3 Mandibular branch: no ocular action.

Injury may cause an anesthetic effect, as occurs in an orbital blow-out fracture

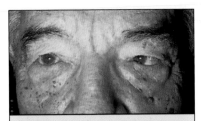

Fig 105 Right lateral rectus paralysis causing an inability to abduct the right eye. Note temporally located light reflex on normal left eye (see Hirscberg's test p. 35, Fig. 97, and Table 5, p. 36.) *Source:* Courtesy of Elliot Davidoff.

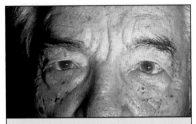

Fig 106 Right lateral rectus paralysis, straight gaze.

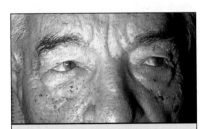

Fig 107 Right lateral rectus paralysis left gaze.

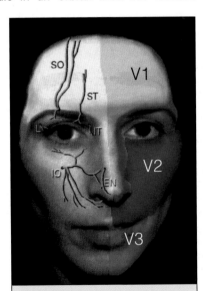

Fig 108 The three divisions of the trigeminal nerve, V1, V2, V3, and the individual nerves. SO, supraorbital; ST, supratrochlear; L, lacrimal; IT, intratrochlear; IO, infraorbital; EN, external nasal.

(Figs 231–233), or pain, as occurs in herpes zoster dermatitis (shingles; Fig. 109) and trigeminal neuralgia (tic douloureux).

Herpes zoster dermatitis (shingles) infects 1 in 3 people in the USA, especially the elderly. It is due to reactivation of the latent varicella virus introduced during an episode of chicken pox in childhood and almost all Americans over age 40 carry this latent virus. Shingles can reoccur, and any symptom could become chronic. It often affects the ophthalmic division of CN V. There may be associated iritis, keratitis, a fever, and adenopathy. Rx: valacyclovir (Valtrex) 1000 mg PO TID × 7 days. It ideally should be started within 72 hours of the onset of skin lesions. The treatment for iritis is similar to the treatment for other causes of iritis. Post-herpetic neuralgia is the most common sequela. The resulting neurotrophic keratitis (Fig. 248) may be treated with an eyedrop, Oxervate, which is structurally identical to the human nerve growth factor. It is used six times a day at 2-hour intervals for 8 weeks. A vaccination, which reduces the incidence and severity of symptoms, is recommended for those over age 50, but is most important in the elderly and immunocompromised. Approximately 20% of patients with ocular involvement may have a chronic course requiring ongoing treatment.

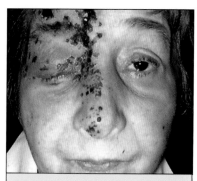

Fig 109 Herpes zoster dermatitis. Think of shingles when the blistering dermatitis follows the distribution of CN V and does not cross the facial midline.

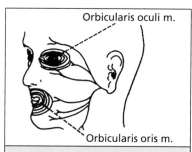

Fig 110 Facial nerve to orbicularis oculi and oris muscles.

Facial nerve (CN VII)

The facial nerve (CN VII) innervates the orbicularis oculi muscle, which closes the lid, and also the muscles that control facial expression (Fig. 110). It also stimulates lacrimal secretion. The common CN VII paralysis in adults is called Bell's palsy and is usually due to ischemia or a virus (Figs 111 and 112). It also serves as sensory nerve to the tongue.

Myokymia refers to minor eyelid spasms of the orbicularis muscle, which the patient senses as a twitching of the muscles of the lid and lasting for seconds or minutes. It usually goes unnoticed by an observer. It may be related to stress, fatigue, caffeine, or hyperthyroidism. Episodes may last for weeks.

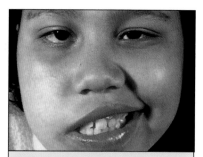

Fig 111 Bell's palsy due to right CN VII paralysis causes incomplete blink, inability to close lids completely and drooping of the lips on that side, especially evident when asked to smile.

Blepharospasm (Figs 110 and 113) is a more severe spasm of the orbicularis muscle causing the eyelids to close involuntarily. It is most commonly a reflex response to ocular surface irritation. The benign essential type has no cause. The first-line treatment is to treat the irritating cause. If this does not help, one may give injections of Botox (onabotulinumtoxin A) into the skin with 5 injections into periorbital muscles involved in closing the lids. It blocks the release of acetylcholine at the neuromuscular junction. Severe cases may require surgical removal of muscle fibers or branches of the seventh nerve. Botox may also be used for muscle spasms such as spastic entropion (Fig. 175). It is also approved by the FDA to treat migraine headaches occurring four or more times a month. In this case, it is injected into the muscles of the forehead above the brow, above the lips and into the chin. It may also be used for cosmetic wrinkles radiating from the lateral corner of the lid (crow's feet).

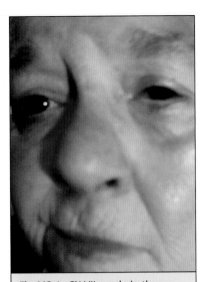

Fig 112 In CN VII paralysis, the inability to close the eye may cause corneal desiccation. To partially remedy this, the left lateral upper and lower tarsus were sutured together (tarsorrhaphy). It may be temporary or permanent.

Vestibulocochlear nerve (CN VIII)

The vestibulocochlear nerve (CN VIII) is the sensory nerve for hearing and balance. The vestibular branch has sensory fibers in the semicircular canals and the vestibule of the inner ear. Their axons connect in a complex system to the nuclei of CN III, IV, and VI in the brainstem, which control the muscles that move the eye. This vestibulo-ocular reflex maintains fixation and balance when the head moves.

Diseases of this pathway cause nystagmus and the illusionary whirling sensation called vertigo. The cochlear division of this nerve is responsible for hearing.

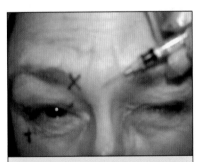

Fig 113 Botox is injected (X) into the orbicularis oculi muscle to treat blepharospasm. Care is taken not to inject the center of the upper lid, which could paralyze the belly of the levator m., resulting in ptosis.

Nystagmus

Nystagmus is an involuntary, rhythmic, to-and-fro movement of the eyes in horizontal, vertical, or rotary fashion. It most commonly occurs at birth or early infancy.

a. Pendular nystagmus has equal motion in each direction.

b. Jerky nystagmus has a quicker movement in one direction than the other.

1 Congenital nystagmus is a pendular nystagmus which may last throughout life. One type of congenital nystagmus is called *spasmus nutans*. This condition may begin at about 6 months of age and often ends at 2 years of age. It may be associated with head nodding. Another type may be due to loss of vision at a young age typically due to albinism or retinal disease. Sometimes, this permanent nystagmus has no obvious cause. It almost always results in some loss of vision by itself.

2 Vestibular nystagmus is a normal response to stimulation of the semicircular canals of the ear, either by rotating the body or placing cold or hot water in the ear. However, it may also be due to diseases of the vestibular system originating in the inner ear or cerebellum. In these cases, it commonly causes new onset of vertigo, i.e., a whirling sensation. A clue in distinguishing vertigo due to ear disease (CN VIII disease) from cerebellar disease is that the latter may also have impairment of speech and gait.

3 Optical kinetic nystagmus is a normal, jerky type of movement as occurs when one watches scenery go by while in a car (Fig. 114).

4 Endpoint gaze nystagmus occurs in certain, often extreme, fields of gaze. It may be caused by medications such as phenytoin (Dilantin) used to treat seizures, and by barbiturates. Neurologic diseases, most commonly multiple sclerosis, ischemic strokes, or brain tumors, should be considered.

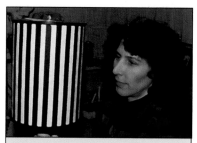

Fig 114 Optokinetic drum that causes optokinetic nystagmus when rotated. Hysterics and malingerers faking total blindness cannot help but move their eyes.

New onset of nystagmus is quite disturbing and warrants a thorough evaluation to determine it's cause. If it is permanent and less in certain fields of gaze (null angle) prisms or infrequently eye muscle surgery may be performed to change the null point to straight ahead gaze

Optic nerve (CN II)

The optic nerve (CN II) is made up of 1.2 million retinal ganglion cell axons which transmit the visual message from the eye to the brain. The nerve begins at the optic disk (papilla) as the ganglion cell axons exit the eye (Figs 115, 335–336, 339, and 343). Each

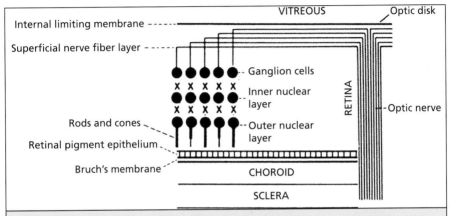

Fig 115 Schematic cross-section of the retina. The ganglion cell fibers on the surface of the retina become covered with a myelin sheath at the optic disk and the continuation of these fibers outside the eye is then called the optic nerve.

fiber picks up a myelin sheath as it exits the eye (Fig. 474) and the whole nerve is covered with a meningeal sheath (pia mater, arachnoid mater, and dura mater) (Fig. 124). The nerve splits at the optic chiasm (Fig. 129 and inside back cover) forming the optic tracts which later synapse in the lateral geniculate body.

When the intraocular ganglion cells or the extraocular optic nerve are damaged, the normal pink or orange optic disk may turn chalk white (Fig. 116).

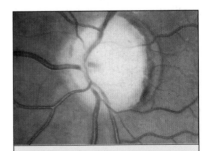

Fig 116 Chalk white optic atrophy resulting from ischemia, transection, toxicity, or inflammation.

In the case of glaucoma, the pallor is associated with excavation (cupping) of the disk (Figs 117 and 340). Another difference is that glaucomatous damage to the optic nerve usually does not cause a decreased pupil response to light and significant loss of color vision as do other causes of optic nerve disease.

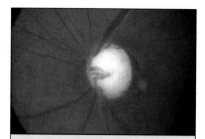

Fig 117 Optic atrophy with cupping due to glaucoma.

Intraocular causes for loss of optic nerve fibers

Glaucoma is a disease of the optic nerve aggravated by high intraocular pressure. It is the most common cause of optic neuropathy. Therefore, a whole chapter is devoted to glaucoma (see Chapter 7).

Retinal ischemia due to retinal artery and vein occlusion or diabetic closure of capillaries may cause loss of ganglion cells and result in pallor of the disk. Thinning of the ganglion cell layer also occurs from elongation of the globe in pathologic myopia, retinitis pigmentosa, chorioretinitis, and numerous less common retinal diseases.

Extraocular causes for loss of optic nerve fibers

When the nerve near the optic disk is inflamed (optic neuritis), you may see papillitis with an ophthalmoscope. Signs of papillitis include flame hemorrhages around the disk, cells in the overlying vitreous, and a blurred disk margin (Fig. 118). Optic neuritis could cause dimming of vision, reduced central vision, decreased pupil reaction to light, reduced color vision, and pain with eye movement.

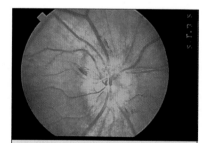

Fig 118 Optic neuritis with papillitis.

When light is shined in a normal eye, both pupils constrict. This is called a consensual light reflex. Damage to the optic nerve (CN II) reduces direct pupillary constriction to light. The diseased eye will constrict well when light shines on the other eye due to the normal consensual reflex. Shining a light back and forth between eyes, called the swinging light test (Fig. 119), reveals the eye with optic disease to be dilating as the light shines on it due to the stronger consensual reflex wearing off. This is called a Marcus Gunn pupil and is helpful in diagnosing optic neuritis. Also, in optic neuritis, the patient claims the light is dimmer in the diseased eye as it is shined back and forth.

Fifty percent of cases of optic neuritis are due to multiple sclerosis. Multiple sclerosis is a chronic relapsing condition with a usual onset between the third and fifth decades and the diagnosis requires a history including multiple sites of involvement. It has a partial genetic and autoimmune etiology that causes multiple areas of demyelination in the central nervous system (Fig. 120). Diplopia due to CN III, IV, or VI paralysis or decreased vision is often the first symptom of the disease. In multiple sclerosis, optic neuritis often occurs without papillitis. The more posterior involvement of the nerve causes more pain on eye movement due to pain fibers in the meningeal sheath covering the nerve. High doses of corticosteroids may shorten the length of time the optic neuritis lasts, but has little effect on the final loss of vision. Diagnosis is supported by an MRI of the brain showing demyelinating plaques (Fig. 120) and a lumbar puncture (spinal tap) in which the cerebral spinal fluid contains more than one band of oligoclonal immunoglobulin proteins.

The next most common cause of optic neuritis is non-inflammatory (nonarteritic) ischemia due to arteriosclerosis. This commonly causes acute unilateral painless loss of vision in older patients—the mean age is 60—and there is no firmly established treatment other than to treat systemic circulatory risk factors. In patients over age 50, ischemia could have an autoimmune cause and one must always consider the possibility of giant cell arteritis (GCA), also called temporal or cranial arteritis (Figs 121–123). Failure to recognize GCA early could result in bilateral blindness and even

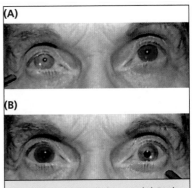

(A)

(B)

Fig 119 Swinging light test. (A) Both pupils constrict when light shines in normal right eye due to consensual reflex. (B) Left pupil in eye with optic neuritis dilates as light shines on it, since consensual stimulation wears off.

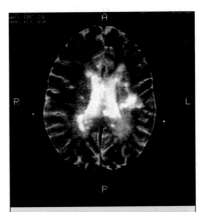

Fig 120 Magnetic resonance imaging (MRI) of the brain. White areas of high intensity correspond to demyelinating plaques, which are present in 90% of known multiple sclerosis cases. MRI of orbit could show thickening of an inflamed optic nerve.

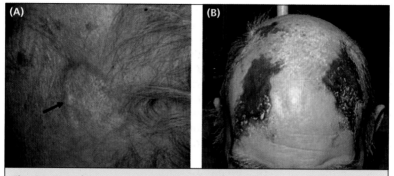

Fig 121 Two of the clinical manifestations of cranial arteritis. (A) Photograph of an enlarged and nodular left temporal artery that is tender to palpation and pulseless. (B) Hemorrhagic necrosis of the scalp in a patient with giant cell arteritis (GCA). *Source:* Campbell et al. *Clin. Experiments Dermatol.*, 2003, Vol. 28, pp. 488–490. Reproduced with permission of Wiley.

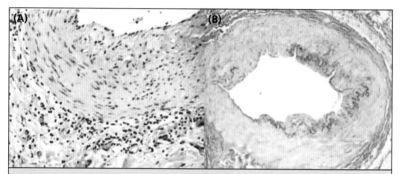

Fig 122 Histopathologic examination of a temporal artery biopsy in a patient with giant cell arteritis (GCA). (A) Hematoxylin and eosin stain shows lymphocytic infiltration of the adventitia. (B) Elastic tissue stain shows fragmentation of the internal elastic lamina and intimal hyperplasia.

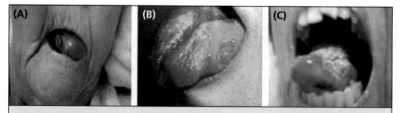

Fig 123 Three examples of ischemic oral lesions caused by giant cell arteritis (GCA). (A) Patient with tongue and lip infarction. (B) Cyanosis and edema in the tongue. (C) A necrotic lesion of the tongue. *Source:* M. Goicochea, J. Correale, L. Bonamico et al., *Headache*, 2007, Vol. 47, pp. 1213–1215. Reproduced with permission of Wiley.

death. The occurrence rises dramatically with each decade. Besides having symptoms typical of optic neuropathy, patients may also have scalp tenderness, pain on chewing, arthritis, weight loss, loss of appetite, and malaise. An elevated erythrocyte sedimentation rate (often over 100) and an elevated C-reactive protein with a positive temporal artery biopsy confirms the diagnosis. Strong suspicion should trigger prompt treatment with high doses of intravenous methylprednisolone—1 gm/day—which should be started even if the biopsy cannot be performed for several days. Then, long-term oral corticosteroids are pre-scribed and adjusted according to patient's signs and symptoms. If corticosteroids are not tolerated, then alternative treatment may include tocilizumab or methotrexate.

Less common causes of optic neuropathy include drug, tobacco, or alcohol toxicity; folic acid or vitamin B_{12} deficiency; and infec-tions such as mumps, measles, influenza, syphilis, tuberculosis, and sarcoidosis. Pressure on the nerve from thyroid orbitopathy, tumors, or elevated intracranial pressure should be considered.

Common brain tumors

Meningioma is a tumor of the three layers of the membranes covering the brain and spinal cord. The outside membrane is called the dura mater; the center is the arachnoid; and the innermost is the pia mater. It is the most common central nervous system tumor and 97% are benign, but 2–3% may be cancerous. They account for 30% of all brain and spinal cord tumors. Optic nerve sheath meningi-omas are often followed with no treatment unless they affect vision (Fig. 124).

Gliomas are tumors arising from cells which surround and support nerve cells. They com-prise 30% of all brain and spinal tumors and 80% are malignant.

The pituitary gland is the size of a pea. Most tumors are benign and referred to as pituitary

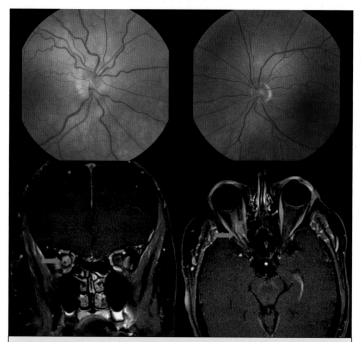

Fig 124 MRI of an optic nerve meningioma with secondary papilledema-like optic disk appearance. Unilateral congestion of the optic disk is due to obstruction of venous outflow from the eye and must be distinguished from papilledema, which is due to elevated intracranial pressure and causes bilateral blurring of disk margins. *Source:* Courtesy of University of Iowa, Eyerounds.org.

adenomas (Figs 81 and 140). They are referred to by the type of hormone they secrete, e.g. adrenocorticotropic (ACTH); growth hormone (GH); prolactin; thyroid stimulating hormone (TSH); reproductive hormones, such as follicle stimulating hormone (FSH); and luteinizing hormone (LH). Non-functioning pituitary tumors produce no hormones and can even suppress normal hormone production resulting in hypopituitarism. About 17 percent of Americans may have this tumor without knowing it. They can rarely become cancerous and are then called pituitary carcinomas.

Idiopathic intracranial hypertension (formally called pseudotumor cerebri) mainly affects young, overweight women of ages 20–40. Cerebrospinal fluid (CSF) pressure on the optic nerve may cause papilledema (Figs

475–478) followed by optic atrophy. Diagnosis is confirmed with CT scan, magnetic resonance imaging (MRI), and lumbar puncture. This spinal tap is positive with CSF pressure greater than 25 cmH$_2$O. Initial treatment includes weight loss, oral acetazolamide, and a low sodium diet. If this conservative treatment is not successful, a shunt from a ventricle in the brain to the peritoneal cavity in the abdomen could lower the pressure. This is often the preferred treatment when headache is the main problem. Incision (fenestration) of the meninges surrounding the ipsilateral optic nerve may shunt CSF into the orbit and is often preferred when there is loss of vision due to pressure on the optic nerve.

The pupil

Both pupils are equally round and approximately 3–4 mm in diameter (Fig. 130). Anisocoria refers to a difference in pupil size, and 4% of normal people may have a difference of as much as 1 mm. Miosis is a constricted pupil, and mydriasis is a dilated pupil. Pupil size is determined by a dilator muscle controlled by the sympathetic nerve and a constrictor muscle that has cholinergic innervation via CN III (Fig. 125 and 130).

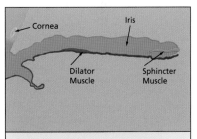

Fig 125 Cross-section of anterior segment showing the iris-corneal junction, and the circular sphincter muscle (green) and radial dilator muscle (blue), which control pupil size. *Source:* Courtesy of Pfizer Pharmaceuticals.

Sympathetic nerve

The iris dilator muscle and Müller's muscle that elevates the lid are both stimulated by the sympathetic nerve that begins in the hypothalamus (Fig. 126) and descends down the spinal column. At C8–T2 it synapses and then exits and passes over the apex of the lung. It ascends in the neck until it synapses, and follows the carotid artery into the skull and orbit. It dilates the pupil in response to the "fight or flight" stimulus. Damage to this nerve causes Horner's syndrome (Fig. 127): miosis, ptosis, and decreased sweating (anhidrosis).

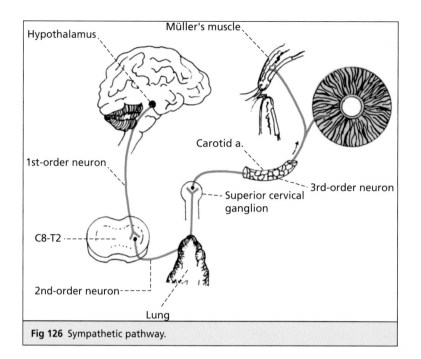

Fig 126 Sympathetic pathway.

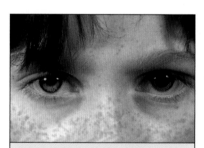

Fig 127 Right Horner's syndrome. Associated neck pain on the same side is highly suggestive of a dissection of the wall of the carotid artery and should be referred immediately to the emergency room for vascular imaging. If caught early, anticoagulation may prevent a stroke (see Fig. 128).

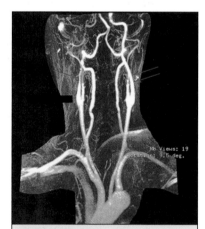

Fig 128 Carotid artery dissection: magnetic resonance angiography (MRA) of right internal carotid (↑) shows decreased blood flow. Left internal carotid artery is normal (↑↑). It commonly follows trauma and is the cause of 25% of strokes in young people (average age 47).

Pupillary light reflex (Fig. 129 and inside back cover)

Light shining on the retina stimulates the optic nerve and then the optic chiasm and optic tract. Here, it exits from the visual pathway to stimulate the Edinger–Westphal nucleus in the midbrain. The pupillary fibers leave the nucleus and travel with CN III until it synapses at the ciliary ganglion in the orbit. It innervates the iris sphincter muscle. Light shining in one eye causes that pupil and the pupil of the other eye to simultaneously constrict. The latter constriction is referred to as the consensual light reflex. Both pupils also constrict when the eye accommodates from distance to near. This normal state may be noted as PERRLA – pupils equally round and reactive to light and accommodation. An MRI of the brain, neck, and upper chest should be considered when Horner's syndrome occurs. In children, rule out neuroblastoma when there are no other obvious causes such as birth trauma.

Pupil irregularities help in determining the severity of brain trauma, strokes and the confirmation of brain stem death. The latter may cause pupil dilation immediately after the event. Then, three hours to four days later, when rigor mortis sets in, the pupils may constrict. Head trauma and strokes are considered more ominous when there are unequal, dilated or constricted pupils. Additionally, the severity is treated with more caution if there is loss of consciousness; lightheadedness; bloody or clear fluid coming from the nose or mouth, with other neurological signs or symptoms.

Addictive recreational drugs cause opposite pupil changes. Opioids such as Fentanyl, codeine and morphine cause miosis, whereas amphetamines ("speed") and also cocaine cause mydriasis.

Adie's pupil (tonic pupil)

This is a dilated pupil with a reduced direct and consensual light reflex. It reacts slowly to accommodation, and eventually becomes smaller and stays smaller than the other eye, hence the name tonic pupil. It is due to a benign defect in the ciliary ganglion (Fig. 129). Resulting denervation hypersensitivity causes the tonic pupil to constrict intensely compared with the other eye in response to one drop of a weak cholinergic, such as pilocarpine 1/10%.

Visual field testing

The field of vision of each eye extends to 170° in the horizontal and 130° in the vertical meridian. Routine testing of vision with a Snellen chart recorded as 20/20 only means that the central 5° corresponding to the fovea and 17° of the macula are normal.

1 Amsler grid. This hand-held black cross-hatched card tests the central 20° of the visual field. Waviness of lines is called metamorphopsia, and is characteristic of a wrinkled retina, which is especially common in wet macular degeneration (Figs 131 and 590; see also Appendix 2).

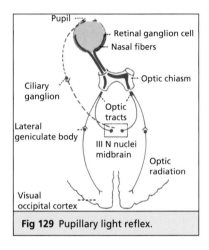

Fig 129 Pupillary light reflex.

Size of pupil	○ 3 ○ 4 ○ 5 ○ 6 ○ 7 ○ 8 ○ 9 ○ 10	
	Miosis	Mydriasis
Constricted (miosis)		Dilated (mydriasis)
Fig 130 Pupillary changes		

Table 6 Causes of small (miotic) and large (mydriatic) pupil (Fig. 125).

Constrictor muscle stimulation	Sympathetic inhibition	Constrictor inhibition	Sympathetic stimulation
↑ *Cholinergic*	↓ *Sympathetic*	↓ *Cholinergic*	↑ *Sympathetic*
Pilocarpine (for glaucoma) Iritis (Fig. 395) CN 111	Horner's syndrome (Figs 126 and 127) Beta-blockers a. for blood pressure atenolol metoprolol b. for glaucoma (Table 11, p. 126) timolol betimol	a. anticholinergic (Table 8, p. 70) todilate thepupil, systemic pills to relieve gastrointestinal and overactive bladder symptoms b. CN III paralysis (Figs 98–100) c. Trauma to sphincter muscle, most often following hyphema (Fig. 369) or high eye pressure greater than 40 mmHg often in narrow angle glaucoma (Fig. 371) d. Adie's pupil	Phenylephrine (to dilate the pupil) Amphetamine (speed) Cocaine Oral or topical decongestants Fight-or-flight Anxiety

2 A tangent screen is a sheet of black felt (Fig. 132). It measures the central 60° of the field. The patient is seated 1 or 2 m from the screen with one eye occluded. The examiner moves a small white ball centrally until the patient first sees it. Areas blind to this small object are tested with progressively larger objects.

3 Hemisphere perimeters (Fig. 133) test the entire 170° of horizontal field and 130° of vertical field. Automated perimeters are expensive, but save examiner's time and give a record of the field. They project increasingly intense stimuli at one location until it is first seen.

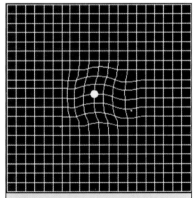

Fig 131 Amsler grid. Distortion in wet macular degeneration.

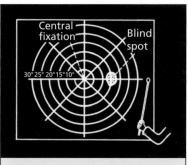

Fig 132 Tangent screen tests the central 60°. It is useful when automated perimetry is too difficult to perform and to monitor enlargement of blind spot in papilledema.

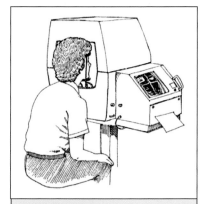

Fig 133 An automated hemisphere perimeter tests central and peripheral fields.

4 Confrontation testing is a less accurate screen used when instruments are not available. The patient is seated opposite the examiner. The patient closes their right eye while the examiner closes his or her left eye. Both fixate on each other's open eye. The examiner moves an object in from the periphery and it should be seen simultaneously by both individuals. This technique compares the patient's and examiner's visual fields.

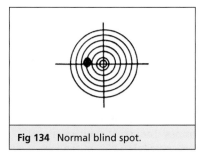

Fig 134 Normal blind spot.

Scotomas due to ocular and optic nerve disease

A scotoma is loss of part of the visual field. Relative scotomas are areas of visual field blind to small objects, but able to perceive larger stimuli. Absolute scotomas are totally blind areas. Scintillating scotomas include sparkling lights (photopsias).

The normal blind spot is an absolute scotoma located 15° temporal to central fixation, which corresponds to the normal absence of rods and cones on the optic disk. It is plotted first (Fig. 134). If the blind spot cannot be located, the validity of the test should be considered.

Central scotomas (Fig. 135) occur in macular degeneration. Central and paracentral scoto-

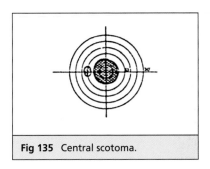

Fig 135 Central scotoma.

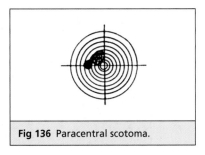

Fig 136 Paracentral scotoma.

mas (Fig. 136) are most characteristic of optic nerve disorders.

Unilateral altitudinal scotomas are defects above or below the horizontal meridian and are most often caused by an occlusion of a superior or inferior retinal artery or vein and retinal detachment (Fig. 137).

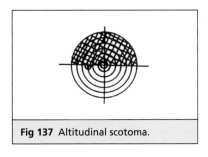

Fig 137 Altitudinal scotoma.

Scotomas due to brain lesions (Fig. 138)

Field defects help to localize the site of brain lesions. Light focused on the temporal retina passes through the optic nerve and stimulates the occipital cortex on the same side, whereas fibers carrying impulses from the nasal retina cross over in the optic chiasm and stimulate

1	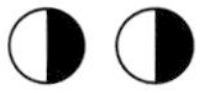 The right homonymous hemianopsia is due to a lesion of the left occipital cortex.
2	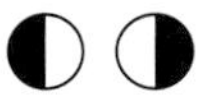 In the optic chiasm the nasal axons from each eye cross over (Fig. 138). Pituitary tumors (Fig. 140) press on these fibers and cause a bitemporal hemianopsia. Since the pituitary is also below the optic chiasm, the inferior-nasal fibers are more often affected. Bilateral superior-temporal defects are, therefore, most common.
3	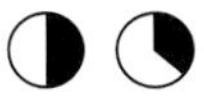 Optic tract lesions cause incongruous hemianopsia; that is, unequal in each eye.
4	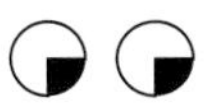 Optic radiation defects are often partial because the fibers are so widespread. A parietal lobe tumor that damages the superior half of the left radiation causes a right homonymous inferior quadrantopsia.
5	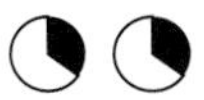 Occipital cortex lesions usually cause a partial homonymous hemianopsia that is often vascular in origin, but tumors, trauma, and abscesses are also common (Figs 81 and 141)

Fig 138 Visual field defects (scotomas) due to brain disease.

the brain on the opposite side (see Fig. 139 and inside back cover). Therefore, defects at or posterior to the chiasm cause loss of vision in both eyes and respect the vertical meridian. If the defects are equal and on the same side, they are called homonymous (see table, notes 1, 4, and 5). If they are unequal on the same side, they are termed incongruous (note 3). If they are on opposite sides in each eye, they are referred to as bitemporal or binasal (note 2).

Color vision

Color vision depends on the ability to see three primary colors: red, green, and blue. Partial defects are inherited in 7% of males and 0.5% of females and are detected using Ishihara or American optical pseudo-isochromatic plates. Loss of color vision could limit one's ability to become an electrician or airline pilot, or follow any profession requiring color discrimination. Acquired color defects may be due to retinal or optic nerve disease, the most common of which is optic neuritis. In acquired cases, test each eye separately and look for differences.

Circulatory disturbances affecting vision

The blood supply to the brain originates from the two carotid arteries in the antero-lateral neck and the two vertebral arteries passing through the cervical vertebrae (refer to Fig. 81 and Table 7, p. 58). The circle of Willis interconnects these four arteries, helping distribute blood to all areas of the brain if one artery is obstructed. Transient loss of vision in persons younger than age 50 is often due to a migrainous spasm of a cerebral artery and occurs in 20% of women and 10% of men. Common triggers may include bright lights and certain foods containing nitrates such as "deli" meats. This may be associated with brief flashes of light resembling zigzag lines (scintillations; Fig. 141) with a headache. It may progress to a homonymous hemianopsia

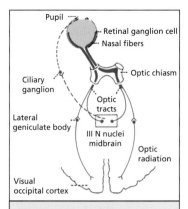

Fig 139 Lesions of the visual pathway (inside back cover). *Source:* Alila Medical Media/Shutterstock.com.

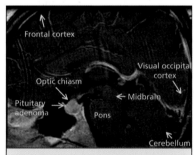

Fig 140 MRI of pituitary adenoma pressing on the optic chiasm, which lies anterior and superior to it. *Source:* Courtesy of Sandip Basak, MD.

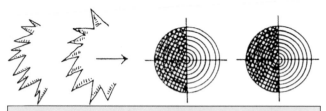

Fig 141 Light flashes called scintillating scotomas are common in migraine. In this case, it progressed to a left homonymous hemianopsia.

lasting for 15–20 minutes. In migraine patients, if neurological symptoms persist for more than 12 hours, especially with non-visual complaints, they should go to an emergency department in a hospital.

In older persons, the transient blurring due to decreased blood flow or heart disease is referred to as a transient ischemic attack (TIA), also called a "ministroke." The attack is caused by cholesterol, fibrin, or calcific emboli being liberated from plaques, in the carotid artery (Figs 81, 143, 582 and 584–586) or from abnormalities in the heart. Symptoms occur as these emboli pass through the eye or visual cortex of the brain and usually last less than a half hour, although the duration could be up to 24 hours. If it lasts longer, it could turn into a permanent obstruction called a stroke.

Five percent of TIAs go on to develop a stroke (cerebrovascular accident, CVA) within a month. So even if the symptoms have already cleared by the time the patient reaches your office, they should be cautioned about the risks of a permanent stroke and advised to see their primary care physician within a short time. If the TIA is still occurring after your examination, they should be sent directly to the emergency room since it could progress to a stroke. Eighty seven percent of strokes are ischemic (Fig. 142) due to emboli or thrombosis and 13% are hemorrhagic often due to a ruptured aneurysm (Figs 81, 101, 102, 144). The latter have a higher risk of fatality. In the emergency room the patient can be thoroughly evaluated to see if they meet the stringent guidelines to receive intravenous tissue

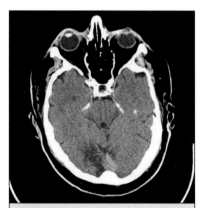

Fig 142 CT scan of right occipital infarct. *Source:* Courtesy of Rand Kirkland, MD.

plasminogen activator (tPA). There is a 3–4.5-hour therapeutic window from the onset of ischemic symptoms to administer this thrombolytic clot busting drug which could increase the chance of recovery from a stroke by 30–50%. A CT scan is usually performed first in the emergency room to be sure it is ischemic and not hemorrhagic. Only then can tPA be safely administered. Be sure the intermittent blurring of vision is not due to dry eyes, which is also common in the elderly.

Tests for decreased circulation

Non-invasive duplex ultrasonography could show carotid stenosis and decreased blood flow. If positive, a CT angiogram may be ordered. Invasive arterial catheter angiography is infrequently used because there is a 1% chance of procedure-related stroke (Fig. 143), but it is still the gold standard. Carotid endarterectomy may be performed in symptomatic (high-risk) patients with 50% narrowing or in asymptomatic patients with 70% stenosis (see Appendix 1, Figs 582–586) (Table 7).

The right and left cavernous sinuses in the brain drain the superior and inferior ophthalmic veins from the orbit and face. Passing through the sinuses are the internal carotid artery, CN III–VI, and the sympathetic nerve (Fig. 144).

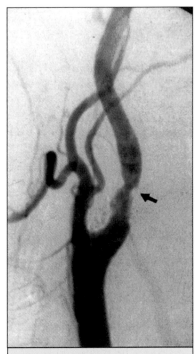

Fig 143 Arteriogram of internal carotid artery narrowing.

Table 7 Visual disturbances due to compromised blood flow (Fig. 81)		
	Carotid circulation	*Posterior cerebral circulation*
Cause	Cardiac abnormalities or carotid atheromas cause emboli to the retina and brain	Neck disorders affecting vertebral artery or emboli from atheroma
Symptoms	Unilateral curtain lasting a few minutes (amaurosis fugax): rarely headache, confusion, contralateral hemiparesis	Hemianopsia in both eyes: usually history of headache, dizziness, diplopia, drop attacks, or ringing in ears
Tests	An audible bruit over carotid artery in neck, duplex ultrasound, CT arteriogram, and cardiac evaluation	CT scan and MRI of brain (Fig. 142) with cardiac evaluation
Rx	Immediate thrombolysis (tPA), anticoagulants, endarterectomy, or stent	Immediate thrombolysis (tPA), anticoagulants, or stent

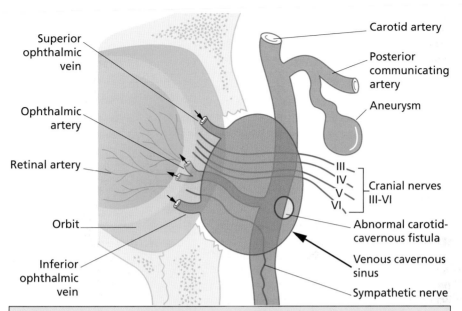

Fig 144 Structures passing through the venous cavernous sinus are the internal carotid artery, CN III–VI, sympathetic nerve, superior and inferior ophthalmic veins, and retinal and ophthalmic arteries. Note the two abnormalities: (1) carotid-cavernous fistula and (2) the posterior communicating artery with its aneurysm pressing on CN III.

Carotid-cavernous fistulas usually result from trauma to an aneurysm of the carotid artery in the cavernous sinus (Figs 144–147). It connects high-pressure arterial to low-pressure venous circulation causing a pulsating exophthalmos with a bruit over the eye, and tortuous—"corkscrew"—conjunctival vessels. Diagnosis is confirmed with carotid arteriography that shows an enlarged superior ophthalmic vein draining in a retrograde way toward the orbit, instead of toward the cavernous sinus.

It must be distinguished from a cavernous sinus thrombosis which causes a non-pulsatile exophthalmos. The latter is often due to infection carried to the sinus via the superior and inferior ophthalmic veins. An MRI is useful to show widening of the cavernous sinus. A carotid-cavernous fistula and a cavernous sinus thrombosis are two causes of exophthalmos that can mimic orbital cellulitis (Figs 226 and 227). What both conditions have in com-

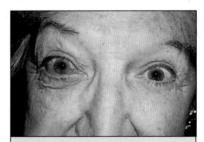

Fig 145 Carotid-cavernous fistula, causing proptosis and dilated cork screw vessels.

mon with orbital cellulitis are conjunctival vascular engorgement and chemosis (Figs 227 and 228); lids that are often swollen shut; and possible involvement of CN III–VI and the sympathetic nerve. Orbital cellulitis is usually unilateral; cavernous sinus thrombosis is commonly bilateral; and carotid-cavernous fistula is unilateral unless there are large connections between the right and left sinuses.

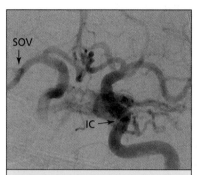

Fig 146 Carotid-cavernous fistula causing bilateral CN VI palsies. Contrast injection into the femoral artery showing an enlarged superior ophthalmic vein (SOV) with retrograde flow and internal carotid artery (IC) within cavernous sinus.

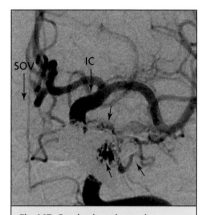

Fig 147 Cerebral angiography through a femoral artery injection and passage of detachable platinum embolization coil through the superior ophthalmic vein located by a cutdown incision near the skinfold of the upper lid. Note the successful clouding of the obliterated cavernous sinus (⊠) due to thrombosis and a narrowed superior ophthalmic vein (SOV) and uninterrupted blood flow through the distal internal carotid artery (IC) as it exits the sinus. *Source:* Courtesy of Stavropoula I. Tjumakaris, MD, and Robert Rosenwasser, MD, Thomas Jefferson University Hospital.

Chapter 4
External structures

The world is governed more by appearances than by realities.

– Daniel Webster

Begin with the four Ls: lymph nodes, lacrimal system, lids, and lashes.

Lymph nodes

Lymphatics from the lateral conjunctiva drain to the preauricular nodes just anterior to the ear. The nasal conjunctiva drains to the sub-mandibular nodes (Fig. 148). Enlarged or tender nodes help to distinguish infectious from allergic lid and conjunctival inflammations.

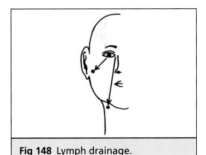

Fig 148 Lymph drainage.

Lacrimal system

With each blink (once every 4 seconds) acting as a lacrimal pump, tears are moved nasally, where they enter the puncta and flow through the canaliculus, lacrimal sac, and the nasolacrimal duct (NLD) into the nose (Fig. 149). All eye drops are more effective and if instilled in the lateral eye and have less systemic side effects if patients press on the puncta and close the eyes for 60 seconds. This minimizes flow into the nose (Figs 150 and 151).

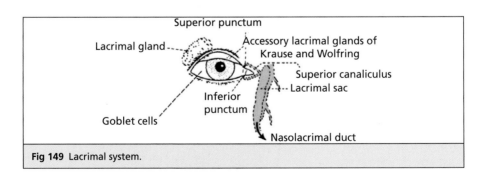

Fig 149 Lacrimal system.

Manual for Eye Examination and Diagnosis, Tenth Edition. Mark W. Leitman.

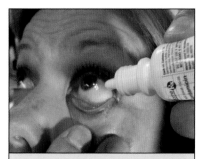

Fig 150 Patients administer one drop by holding the bottle like a pencil with one hand while the other hand pulls lower lid down as they look up. It is even easier if the patient lies down to stabilize the head, but some prefer to look in a mirror.

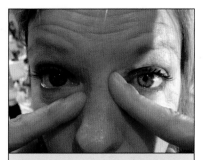

Fig 151 After administering the drop, have the patient push on the upper and lower punctum for 60 seconds. This minimizes systemic side effects from the drug entering the nose and maximizes eye contact. Ask patients to show you their technique. The picture demonstrates the correct technique on the left side.

The tear film is made up of an outer oily component, a middle watery layer, and a deep mucous layer (Fig. 152). A decrease in the oily, mucous, or watery tear could cause symptoms such as dryness, stinging, grittiness, sore eyes, blurry vision, and tearing from irritations. Dry eye disease (DED) is reported to affect 5% of the general population, 9% of menopausal women, and 34% of the elderly. With most external eye infections, the tear film is highly infectious. In AIDS, only bloody tears are so far considered infectious. In any case, wash your hands between patient examinations.

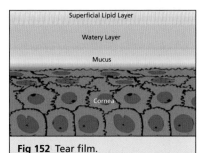

Fig 152 Tear film.

The oily, superficial layer is secreted by the meibomian glands in the upper and lower lids (Fig. 153) and prevents desiccation and lubricates the eyelids as they pass over the globe. Dysfunction of these glands occurs in almost half of Americans and often manifests with a toothpaste-like discharge (Fig. 154) with occasional infection, referred to as *posterior blepharitis*. It is the most common reason for dry eye disease. In my practice, not a day goes by without seeing patients with blepharitis.

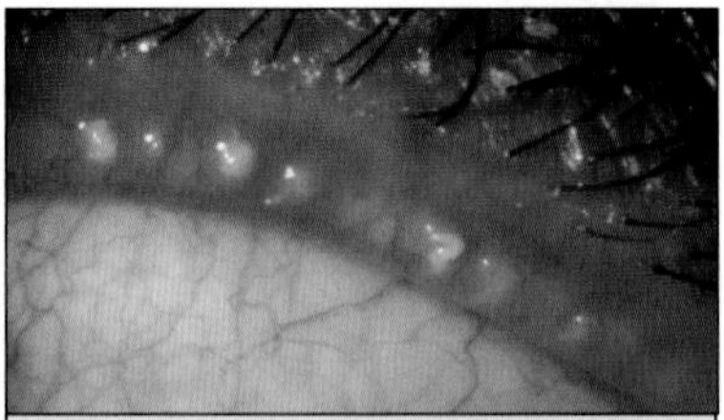

Watery tears provide anti-infective defenses, wash away debris, and smooth surface irregularities. Seventy percent is tonically secreted by the accessory lacrimal glands of Krause and Wolfring in the conjunctiva (Fig. 149). The lacrimal glands' (Fig. 149) contribution to watery

Fig 154 Meibomian glands in both the upper and lower lid that normally secrete a clear, oily meibum. In this case, the glands are dysfunctional with a white, pasty discharge. *Source*: Courtesy of Michael Lemp, MD.

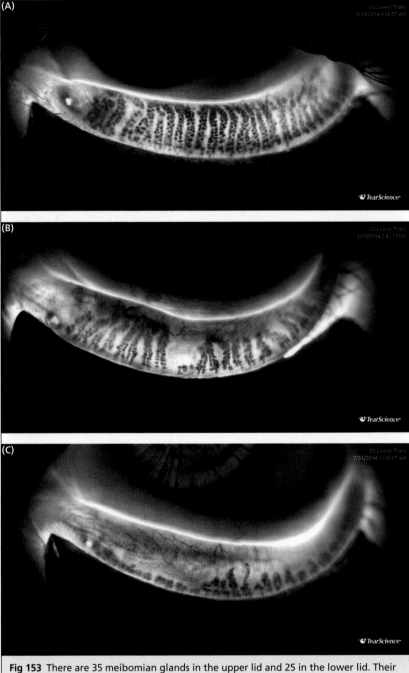

Fig 153 There are 35 meibomian glands in the upper lid and 25 in the lower lid. Their dysfunction is the most common reason for dry eye and ocular surface infections. They are demonstrated with transillumination of lid margin (meibography) showing meibomian glands: (A) normal; (B) localized dropout; (C) severe dropout. *Source*: Courtesy of LipiView II with DMI, TearScience.

tears is mostly a reflex response to emotion and ocular irritations. The corneal reflex arc has the trigeminal nerve (CN V) as its afferent pathway and the facial nerve as the efferent branch. Damage to the sensory CN V nerves can cause dry eye and other ocular surface changes (neurotrophic keratitis). It may result from LASIK and PRK surgery, diabetes, and herpes simplex or zoster keratitis. Damage to the efferent CN VII, as in Bell's palsy, causes desiccation due to incomplete blink reflex and inability to close the eye completely, especially at night. Corneal sensitivity (CN V) may be tested by touching a sterile cotton tip applicator to each eye and comparing blink reflexes. A wide variety of medications reduce watery tear production. They include diuretics and beta-blockers used to treat blood pressure, tranquilizers, antidepressants, antihistamines, anti-Parkinson disease drugs, bladder anti-spasmotics, and gastroprotective and gastric motility agents. A decrease in the watery or mucous component could be due to aging or inflammation associated with systemic auto-immune diseases such as Sjögren's disease (dry eye, dry mouth, and arthritis). The resulting inflammatory ocular surface epithelial disease is called *keratoconjunctivitis sicca*. Fifty percent of Sjögren's patients have rheumatoid arthritis or lupus, both of which may also cause dry eye independent of Sjögren's. All three of these autoimmune diseases are often treated with hydroxychloroquine.

Mucous is secreted by goblet cells which account for 5–20% of the conjunctival cells. The mucous traps exfoliated cells, bacteria, and other foreign bodies and washes them into the nose. Goblet cells decrease after menopause; or from any condition that damages the conjunctiva, such as Stevens–Johnson syndrome (Fig. 10), ocular pemphigoid (Fig. 303 and 304), trachoma (Fig. 308), alkali burns (Figs 254 and 255), or vitamin A deficiency (Fig. 155). The latter could cause dysfunction of the conjunctival epithelial cells (Fig. 240) reducing both tears and mucous. Vitamin A deficiency could be due to poor diet or malabsorption which is surging due to the popularity of gastric bypass surgery used to treat obesity. Loss of

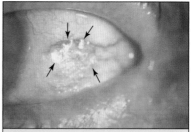

Fig 155 A white Bitot's spot (↑) is due to conjunctival keratinization from vitamin A deficiency. These lesions appear in the perilimbal area. *Source*: Ahad, M., Puri, P., Chua, C. et al. Bitot's spots following hemicolectomy. *Eye*, Vol. 17, pp. 671–673 (2003). https://doi.org/10.1038/sj.eye.6700427

vision from vitamin A deficiency may result from desiccation of the cornea due to dryness or from decreased function of the rod receptors in the retina, which requires this vitamin to produce the visual pigment rhodopsin. Paradoxically, excess vitamin A is toxic and can cause elevated intracranial pressure with loss of vision (Figs 475–478).

Dry eye may cause intermittent haziness of the cornea resulting in transient blurring of vision. This blur must be distinguished from the transient ischemic attacks (TIAs—ministrokes) especially in seniors who may be predisposed to both conditions.

The diagnosis of DED may be confirmed by seeing punctate haziness of corneal epithelial cells (Figs 156, 248, and 249) and fluorescein

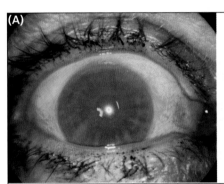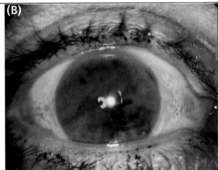

Fig 156 Tear breakup time (TBUT). (A) Fluorescein placed on a normal cornea and observed with cobalt blue light has a uniform appearance. (B) With the lids held open, the pattern may abnormally break up before 10 seconds. *Source*: Courtesy of Elliot Davidoff, MD.

staining of underlying stroma when illuminated by cobalt blue light. The integrity of the tear film layer is estimated by testing tear breakup time (TBUT) (Fig. 156). The Schirmer test measures tears on the surface of the eye. A drop of anesthetic is instilled, and a strip of folded filter paper is placed on the surface of the conjunctiva (Fig. 157). Less than 10 mm of moist paper in 5 minutes is presumptive of a dry eye. Patients with dry eye have an abnormal Schirmer test 21% of the time, corneal staining with fluorescein 50% of the time,

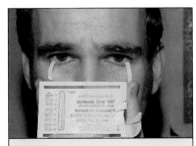

Fig 157 Schirmer test.

conjunctival staining with lissamine green, and an abnormal TBUT in 60% of cases. Lissamine green specifically stains devitalized conjunctival epithelium (Fig. 158).

Dry eye is treated in the daytime with artificial tears and at night with ointments. There are many on the market and vary mostly by their viscosity, cost, and whether they have preservatives. Viscous agents, especially ointments, maximize duration of action but interfere with vision and are therefore preferred during sleep. Symptoms of dry eye are more common in eyes that do not close at night, as with lagophthalmos (Fig. 251); Bell's palsy (Fig. 111); Grave's disease (Figs 1 and 177); and ectropion (Fig. 174). It is further aggravated by those with sleep apnea due to chronic obstructive lung disease using a continuous positive airway pressure (CPAP) that might blow on their eye. Unfortunately, the effect of lubricating drops may last less than an hour, often leading to excessive use. Benzalkonium chloride (BAK)—the most common preservative in most eye drops—could cause surface toxicity, especially in glaucoma patients using other drops. Preservative-free (PF) drops in individual ampules are then indicated. If annoying symptoms persist, the puncta may be closed with absorbable or permanent punctal plugs (Figs 159 and 160). If temporary plugs are shown to improve chronic symptoms, the

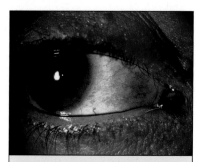

Fig 158 Lissamine green stain of devitalized conjunctival epithelial cells. The density of stain increases in dry eye and is usually in the interpalpebral area. *Source*: Courtesy of Eric Donnenfeld, MD, NYU Medical Center.

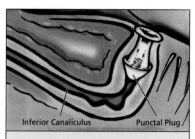

Inferior Canaliculus   Punctal Plug

Fig 159 Punctal plug. Problems include 40% loss of plugs, 9% epiphora, and 10% ocular irritation, especially from the inability to flush toxic and inflammatory chemicals from the surface of the eye. *Source:* Courtesy of Eagle Vision.

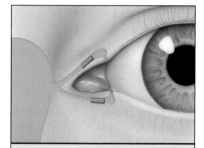

Fig 160 Absorbable punctal plugs—no larger than a grain of rice—may be inserted deeper into the tear duct preventing extrusion. *Source*: Courtesy of FCI Ophthalmics.

puncta may be permanently closed with a cautery. Room humidifiers may be tried, and oral flaxseed oil (1000 mg BID) may increase meibomian gland secretions. Computer use and reading suppress blinking, and desiccation of surface tears aggravates DED. Intentional blinking during computer use should be encouraged. Restasis (cyclosporine ophthalmic emulsion) or Xiidra (lifitegrast) eye drops reduce inflammation of tear producing cells and either can be used twice a day to increase tear production by suppressing lymphocyte T-cell-induced inflammation. Low dose steroid eye drops, such as fluorometholone (FML, 0.19%) are infrequently added. DED may cause corneal changes, resulting in fluctuating vision. It is critical to document its presence before corneal refractive or cataract surgery, which could aggravate the condition and thus cause patient disgruntlement. The intermittent blurring should not be confused with circulatory disturbances in older patients.

Tearing (epiphora)

Tearing is a very common complaint and is often minor enough so as not to require the workup and treatment discussed below.

There are two causes of tearing (epiphora):

1 increased tear production due to emotion and eye irritation; paradoxically, dry eye stimulates reflex tearing;
2 tears that are produced normally but which cannot flow properly into the nose.

Tearing due to failure of drainage system

Once increased tear production is ruled out as the cause of tearing, an evaluation is made of the patency of the ducts leading into the nose. An obstruction is presumed if fluorescein dye placed on the conjunctiva (Fig. 161) disappears slowly and asymmetrically from one eye, or runs over the lid onto the cheek.

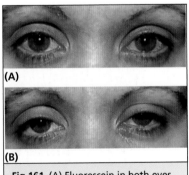

Fig 161 (A) Fluorescein in both eyes. (B) Obstruction prevents exit of dye in left eye.

Failure of the tear to reach the puncta

This could be due to horizontal laxity of the lower lid which decreases the pumping action of the blink reflex, or an everted puncta, as occurs in an ectropion (Fig. 174), in which case the tear lake is not in contact with the punctal orifice. Either can often be corrected by surgically tightening the lower lid with a full-thickness wedge resection.

Obstruction at the puncta or canaliculus

The puncta may become narrowed due to aging, topical drugs, trauma, and infections, especially from blepharitis.

The puncta and canaliculi can be dilated with progressively wider-diameter punctal probes (Fig. 162). If the lumen is still inadequate, a snip incision can widen the puncta. If still unsuccessful, a self-retaining bicanalicular stent (Fig. 163) can be inserted in the office with topical anesthetic and left in place for 3 months. If epiphora is primarily due to canalicular failure, a Pyrex glass tube may be permanently inserted, creating a fistula from the conjunctiva to the nasal cavity. Traumatic laceration of the canaliculus can be repaired using a pigtail probe (Figs 162C and 164). The probe is passed through the upper puncta

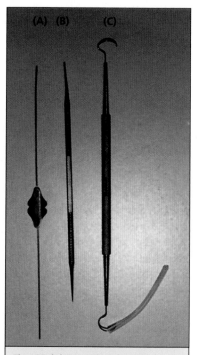

Fig 162 (A) Punctal probe. (B) Punctum dilator. (C) Pigtail probe.

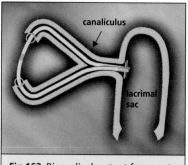

Fig 163 Bicanalicular stent for puncta stenosis or canalicular constriction. *Source*: Courtesy of FCI Ophthalmics.

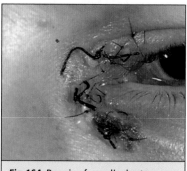

Fig 164 Repair of canalicular tear.

toward the laceration. A silicone tube is threaded onto it and is withdrawn. The probe is then passed through the lower puncta and the other end of the silicone tube is threaded onto it and is withdrawn, forming a continuous lumen to heal over the tube.

Rarely, the canaliculus can be obstructed due to an *Actinomyces israelii* infection. In this case, incise the canaliculus and remove sand-like concretions. This bacterium is sensitive to penicillin and sulfa drugs.

Tearing due to NLD obstructions

In adults, obstructions result from chronic nasal inflammation. In infants, the distal opening of this duct in the nose—called the valve of Hasner—fails to open at birth, in 1 of 9 newborns. Although 90% spontaneously open by 1 year of age, repeated infections may mandate treatment at 6–12 months. In these infants, the puncta may be irrigated and/or probed to the nose (Figs 165 and 166). The same technique can be used in adults. If it is still narrowed, a balloon catheter may be used to widen the passage (Fig. 167), and/or a silicone stent may be inserted through the puncta, canaliculus, and the NLD into the nose and left in place for 2–4 months.

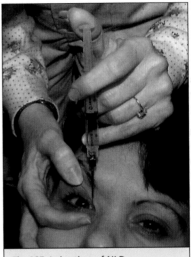

Fig 165 Irrigation of NLD.

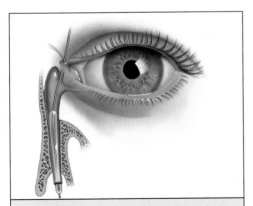

Fig 167 Balloon catheter dacryoplasty: inflate the balloon with sterile saline. *Source:* Courtesy Quest Medical, Inc.

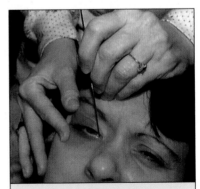

Fig 166 Probing of NLD for congenital obstruction is successful 77% of the time after the first attempt and 90% after the second.

If it still remains closed, a new surgical opening in the nasal bone is created and the mucosa of the lacrimal sac is sutured to the nasal mucosa (dacryocystorhinostomy) (DCR). Besides tearing, an additional motivation for performing the latter surgical procedure is recurring infections of the lacrimal sac (dacryocystitis; Fig. 168), caused by stagnant tear flow. A surgical DCR is 85% successful.

Signs of dacryocystitis are swelling and tenderness over the lacrimal sac with pus exuding from the puncta when pressure is applied to the sac. Rx: massage the sac, nasal decongestant, local (see Table 8) and systemic

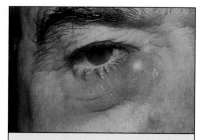

Fig 168 Dacryocystitis.

Table 8 Common topical anti-infectives.

Betadine (Povidone-Iodine 0.5%—Applied topically to the eye for 2 minutes before most intraocular surgeries. It has a broad-spectrum impact. Reportedly, it kills 85% of surface bacteria in that time.

Hypochlorous acid 0.02%—An over-the-counter antiseptic (used on lid margin) to treat blepharitis. Normally secreted by white blood cells to combat infection; similar to an ingredient in "Clorox" and additives to swimming pools. It kills 99% of bacteria in 30 seconds.

Topical antibiotics

Polytrim (Polymyxin B, trimethoprim)—An inexpensive, generic broad-spectrum drop used to treat commonly occurring bacterial conjunctivitis. Especially popular with pediatricians, it is used to treat pseudomonas and some methicillin resistant staphylococcal aureus (MRSA).

Ciloxin (ciprofloxacin) and Ocuflox (ofloxacin)—Both are inexpensive, generic broad-spectrum fluroquinolones and they are often a first-line choice for commonly occurring bacterial conjunctivitis and blepharitis. Resistance with repeated use is a problem.

Besivance (besifloxocin)—A more expensive broad-spectrum fluroquinolone topically used for pre- and post-op surgeries and vision-threatening corneal ulcers. One advantage is it has never been used systemically so there is less resistance.

Vigamox (moxifloxacin)—A broad-spectrum fluoroquinolone drop with no preservative used topically and also could be injected into the anterior chamber in cataract surgery to prevent endophthalmitis.

Tobrex (tobramycin) and Gentac (gentamycin)—Both are generic aminoglycosides and less expensive with broad-spectrum action.

Sulfacetamide 10% is bacteriostatic inexpensive generic used less often as an alternative to previous cidal drops, if allergy or resistance develops to them.

Available as generic ointments are bacitracin 500 units/gm, erythromycin 0.3%, sulfacetamide 10%, tobrex 0.3%, and ciprofloxacin 0.3%. They are preferred for nighttime use since they blur vision and for treating lid margin infections such as blepharitis, sties, and infected chalazions.

Topical antivirals

Viroptic (trifluridine 1%)—A generic commonly used to treat herpes keratitis.

Zirgan gel (ganciclovir)—A more expensive branded antiviral alternative to Viroptic for treating herpes keratitis. It has less corneal toxicity and is used five times a day.

---

the base is indicated if it recurs since it rarely may harbor a carcinoma.

Phakomatoses

Four congenital syndromes that include lesions of the brain, skin, and eye are called phakomatoses. The early onset of skin lesions in these infants and young children provide a red flag to alert one to other problems.

1 Tuberous sclerosis is a condition appearing in the first 3 years of life. Patients may manifest seizures, mental deficiency, and sebaceous adenoma. Seventy five percent die before age 20 (Figs 197 and 198).

2 Sturge–Weber syndrome includes facial port wine capillary malformations (Fig. 199) and

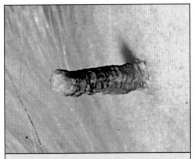

Fig 196 Cutaneous horn.

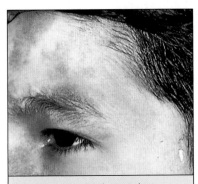

Fig 199 Sturge–Weber syndrome.

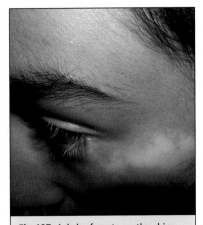

Fig 197 Ash-leaf spots on the skin are multiple, depigmented macules with irregular borders. They are usually the first sign of tuberous sclerosis and appear in up to 90% of patients.

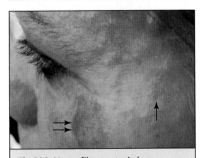

Fig 200 Neurofibromatosis (von Recklinghausen disease) is characterized by neurofibromas of the skin (↑) and nervous system, and café-au-lait spots (↓↓), which are irregularly shaped brown macules. There are usually multiple (five or more) increasing in size from 0.5 to 1.5 cm in adults.

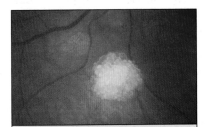

Fig 198 Retinal astrocytoma in tuberous sclerosis. Areas of calcification give mulberry appearance. *Source*: Courtesy of Dana Gabel, Barnes Retinal Institute, St. Louis, MO.

mental retardation in half of the patients. They should be monitored for early onset glaucoma or choroidal and central nervous system (CNS) hemangiomas. Intraocular surgery should be approached with caution since serious hemorrhage with loss of eye could occur.

3 Neurofibromatosis is a condition that is inherited in an autosomal dominant pattern with incomplete penetrance. Tumors could affect the optic nerve, iris, retina, and skin of the lid (Fig. 200). Lisch nodules in the iris are present in 94% of patients (Fig. 201). Brown macular skin lesions occur early on and eventually in 99% in patients.

4 von Hippel-Lindau syndrome is a rare (1:36,000) inherited condition (Figs 202 and 203). Hemangiomas of the retina and iris could cause retinal detachments and glaucoma. Ocular anomalies should alert one to lesions elsewhere on the skin or in the brain.

Leprosy is a chronic disease caused by acid-fast *Mycobacterium leprae*. It is probably transmitted by the respiratory route and usually involves prolonged exposure in childhood (Figs 204 and 205).

Anterior and posterior blepharitis

Blepharitis refers to inflammation or infection of the lid margin. It is extremely common

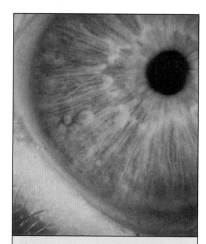

Fig 201 Lisch nodules on the iris of a patient with neurofibromatosis. *Source*: Courtesy of S.J. Charles, FRCS, and *Arch. Ophthalmol.*, Nov. 1989, Vol. 107, p. 1572. Copyright 1989, American Medical Association.

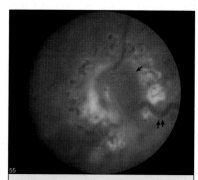

Fig 202 von-Hipple-Lindau syndrome: Hemangioblastoma of retina ↑ with dilated feeder vessel ↑↑. The eye findings are often the first sign of this disease. It presents in the first three decades of life. *Source*: Courtesy of University of Iowa, Eyerounds.org.

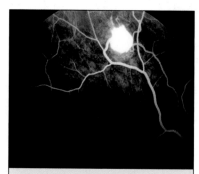

Fig 203 Fluorescein angiogram of hemangioblastoma. *Source*: Courtesy of Stuart Green, MD.

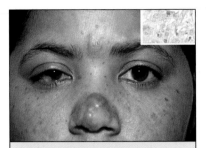

Fig 204 A 22-year-old from Cape Verde Islands with lepromatous leprosy. There are macular and erythematous nodular lesions on face, trunk, and extremities. Fite's stain/acid-fast bacilli in skin biopsy confirms the diagnosis.

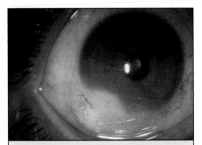

Fig 205 Leprosy causing a solid nodule on the ocular surface together with granulomatous iritis. *Source*: Courtesy of Carly Seidman, BS, and *Arch. Ophthalmol.*, Dec. 2010, Vol. 128, p. 1522. Copyright 2010, American Medical Association. All rights reserved.

and is reported to occur in up to 50% of adults. There is rarely a day that goes by that an eye doctor does not treat it or one of its sequelae, such as conjunctivitis, sties, chalazia, corneal ulcers, lid cellulitis, dry eye, or intolerance to contact lenses.

Infections of the cornea, conjunctiva, and lid margins can usually be treated with relatively inexpensive generic antibiotic eye drops and ointments (see Table 8 p. 70). A lot of thought has gone into giving brand medications short, easy-to-remember names without having to write all components and concentrations. Writing these brand names, and approving the generic form on the prescription pad, saves time and increases accuracy.

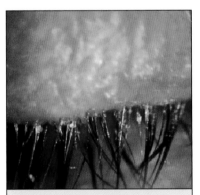

Fig 206 Anterior blepharitis with crusting flakes on lashes. *Source*: Courtesy of Michael Lemp, MD.

Anterior blepharitis manifests with crusting, redness, and ulcerative lesions around the lashes (Figs 206–208). Infections are usually due to staphylococcal bacteria. The seborrheic type, associated with dandruff of the scalp and eyebrows, responds to appropriate shampoos.

A less common type is caused by the *Demodex* mite (demodex blepharitis). This member of the spider family inhabits the lashes of almost all adults. Some people are more sensitive and get itching and conjunctivitis. It can be

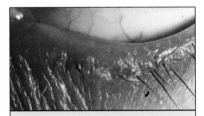

Fig 207 Anterior blepharitis with crusting and ulcerative lesions around lashes. *Source*: Courtesy of Michael Lemp, MD.

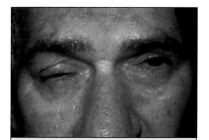

Fig 208 Blepharoconjunctivitis in acne rosacea. This chronic condition is associated with engorged vessels and pustules on the nose, forehead, cheeks, and chin.

detected at the slit lamp by noting cylindrical cuffs around the base of the lashes (Fig. 209). There are commercial tea tree preparations available (Cliradex and Demodex®) to treat this infestation.

Posterior blepharitis (Figs 153,154 and 210–213) may involve all meibomian glands on both the upper and lower lids. These glands often become dysfunctional, losing their ability to produce the meibum which contributes the oily portion of the tear film (Figs 152 and 153). It has been reported that up to 86% of dry eyes are due in part to this disorder. It is often associated with acne rosacea (Fig. 208). White heads on the meibomian orifices (Fig. 210)

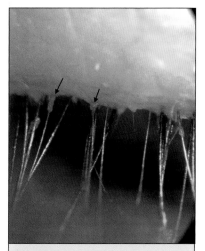

Fig 209 Demodex blepharitis is identified by a telltale cylindrical cuff around the base of eyelash (↑). Compare with pediculosis capitus, which is a different lid infestation in which the parasite and eggs (nits) are seen at slit lamp (Fig. 185). *Source*: Courtesy of Eric Donnenfeld, MD, NYU Medical Center.

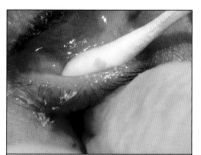

Fig 211 Posterior blepharitis: dysfunctional meibomian glands may be diagnosed by massaging the lid and revealing a toothpaste-like secretion. It is also therapeutic.

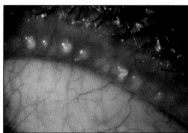

Fig 210 Toothpaste-like meibum spontaneously exuding from glands make for an easy diagnosis. *Source*: Courtesy of Eric Donnenfeld, MD, NYU Medical Center.

and foamy residue (Fig. 212) are abnormal clues.

Anterior and posterior blepharitis often occur together (Fig. 213). Both require good lid hygiene, including warm soaks and mechanical scrubs for which over-the-counter cleaning solutions are available. Less expensive baby shampoo may be used and closed-eye rinsing of lashes in shower is recommended. These conditions are often chronic, and maintenance of preventive therapy between attacks should be encouraged.

For more resistant cases involving recurrent infections, commercially available lid-margin solutions containing hypochlorous acid (0.02%) are available over-the-counter or by prescription. It is the same anti-microbial also present in "Chlorox bleach" and secreted internally as part of the human body's natural defense. It kills 99.9% of bacteria. Antibiotic drops or ointment may be added (see Table 8, p.70). Nonsteroidal anti-inflammatory drugs (NSAIDs), such as ketorolac 0.5%, are sometimes needed (Table 14, p. 145). Steroids may be added with caution, since gritty, sore eyes with fluorescein staining of the cornea are common to both blepharitis and herpes keratitis. Herpes can be made worse with steroids.

An oral antibiotic is added to treat more severe bacterial conditions such as lid cellulitis (Fig. 217); corneal ulcers (Figs 261–263), especially central; or keratitis (Fig. 248) unresponsive to topical treatment. Oral doxycycline 20 or 100 mg BID is often preferred since it kills bacteria that produce lipase. This enzyme causes a breakdown of the meibum lipid secretions that lubricate the eye. The resulting soap-like residues may produce pathognomonic bubbles on the lid margin (Fig. 212).

The lid margin may be massaged to reveal a diagnostic white paste, instead of the usual clear oil. The patient should be told that this sometimes uncomfortable procedure is also therapeutic (Fig. 211). Many get significant relief and return at regular intervals requesting massage.

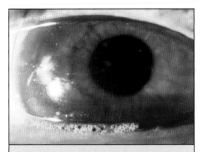

Fig 212 Posterior blepharitis with foamy residue overlying the meibomian glands. *Source*: Courtesy of Michael Lemp, MD.

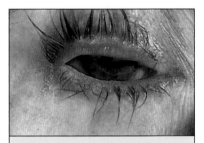

Fig 213 Anterior and posterior blepharitis often occur together.

Chalazia (Fig. 214) are cystic enlargements of the meibomian glands that occur due to the clogging of an orifice. Retention of lipid and its breakdown by-products incite a granulomatous inflammatory reaction. They are usually painless, unless infected. As with blepharitis, treatment includes warm compresses and lid scrubs. Antibiotic/steroid drops (see Table 8, p. 70 and Table 14, p. 145), or even intralesional steroid injections, with or without antibiotic, are often considered. Oral generic doxycycline with incision and drainage are sometimes needed (Figs 214 and 215).

Sties are infections of the glands of Zeis and Moll around the lashes (Fig. 216). These pimples are treated with hot soaks, local antibiotics, and incision. Systemic antibiotics are indicated if there is significant surrounding cellulitis.

Lid cellulitis is a diffuse infection often due to a sty, chalazion, bug bite, or cut. Lids are red and tender (Fig. 217). There may be adenopathy and fever. Rx: topical and systemic antibiotics. Shriveled skin is an initial indication that lid cellulitis is responding to treatment. Be cautious. When severe, it can penetrate the orbital septum (see Fig. 218), resulting in orbital cellulitis (Figs 226 and 227) that could extend into the brain, causing meningitis and even death.

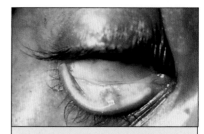

Fig 214 Chalazia point internally.

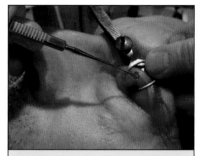

Fig 215 A chalazion clamp is used to minimize bleeding during incision and curettage.

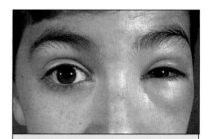

Fig 217 Preseptal cellulitis – i.e., in front of orbital septum (Fig. 218) – typically affects children and is usually secondary to lid infections. Orbital cellulitis most often originates from infections behind the orbital septum, most commonly in the sinuses (Figs 224–227).

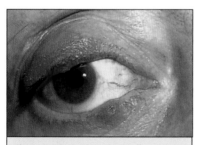

Fig 216 Sties point externally.

Chapter 5
The orbit

Burglars know there's more than one way to skin a vault.

– James Chiles

The orbit is a cone-shaped vault (Figs 218 and 221). At its apex are three orifices through which pass the nerves, arteries, and veins supplying the eye.

Imaging

Unlike the eye, in which most parts are amenable to direct visualization, evaluation of the orbit often requires the use of diagnostic tools such as CT scans (Figs 2, 3, 142, 224, 225, 227–229B, 234, 402, and 480) and

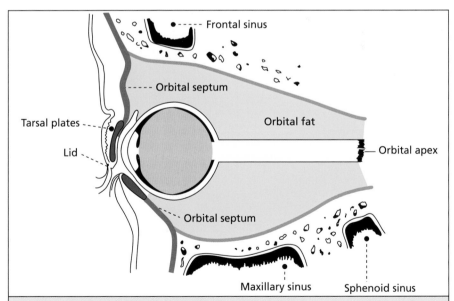

Fig 218 Side view of orbit; periosteum (periorbital) of the orbit (green), the orbit septum (red), and tarsal plate (blue) are continuous connective tissue membranes. This fibrous membrane then goes on to cover the optic nerve as it exits the orbit and is continuous with the dura mater covering the brain.

MRI (Figs 120, 124, and 140). CT scans are usually the radiologic technique of choice to evaluate orbital diseases such as fracture (Fig. 231), foreign bodies, thyroid disease (Figs 2 and 3), and sinusitis (Figs 223 and 224). MRIs are preferred for soft tissue and neurologic conditions (Fig. 124).

CT scanning has made amazing contributions to medical diagnosis, but it is a large contributor to the six-fold increase in diagnostic radiation in the last 30 years, because of overutilization. It is predicted that CT scans may be responsible for 1.5–2.0% of all future cancers in the USA and studies reveal that patients are not informed of this risk 90–95% of the time. Special caution should be given to children and pregnant women. Contrast materials are preferred for most CT and MRI procedures since it increases sensitivity. Usage of iodine-based chemicals used in CT scans should be minimized with histories of iodine allergy and in pregnant women and children. MRI is more hazardous with foreign bodies of unknown origin and in pregnant women and patients with pacemakers, metallic cardiac valves, and other ferro-magnetic implants. Gadolinium is used for contrast.

Vascular testing may be done with CT or MRI angiography (Figs 128, 146, and 147). CT-A can detect 3–5 mm cerebral aneurysms and venous thrombosis. Either CT-A or MR-A is used to detect carotid artery stenosis.

The yellow orbital fat may herniate through the orbital septum under the conjunctiva (Fig. 219) and shouldn't be mistaken for an abnormal growth.

The fat more commonly herniates under the skin of the lower lid. The apparent swelling shouldn't be confused with lid edema. Unlike fluid, the fat may be rolled beneath the examiner's fingertips (Figs 173 and 220).

Sinusitis

The orbit is surrounded on four sides by the periorbital paranasal sinuses, i.e., the maxillary, frontal, sphenoid, and ethmoid sinuses.

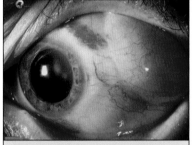

Fig 219 Yellow subconjunctival fat. *Source:* Courtesy of University of Iowa, Eyerounds.org

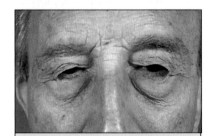

Fig 220 Subcutaneous orbital fat often causes a desire for cosmetic excision, but caution patient about the risk of orbital hemorrhage (Fig. 235).

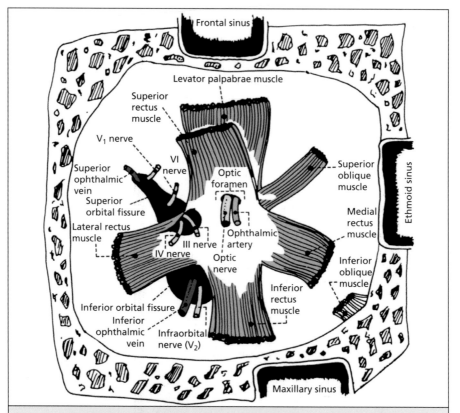

Fig 221 Front view shows the apex of the orbit. Note proximity to sinuses with its potential for causing infection and the significant number of blood vessels vulnerable to hemorrhage (Fig. 235).

Pain, described as deep, or behind the eye, is most often due to allergy or infection of these sinuses. Pressure applied to the skin overlying the inflamed frontal, maxillary, and ethmoidal sinuses may cause tenderness (Fig. 223). The sphenoid sinus is behind the globe and cannot be tested in this way (Fig 222).

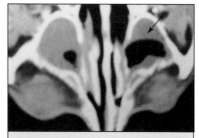

Fig 222 CT scan of sphenoid sinusitis with air-fluid level (↑).

Clues that may indicate disease of the orbit

1 Proptosis (exophthalmos): forward bulging of the eye (Fig. 1).
2 Enophthalmos: sunken eye (Fig. 230).

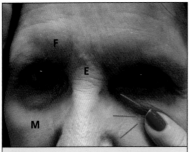

Fig 223 One piece of evidence for the diagnosis of sinusitis is to elicit tenderness by palpating over the frontal (F), ethmoid (E), or maxillary (M) sinus. In this case, the left maxillary sinus is involved.

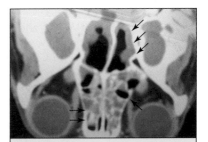

Fig 224 CT showing three typical findings of ethmoiditis. A level flat surface of fluid accumulation (↑) and opacification of the air spaces (↑↑) are common in an acute process. Thickening of mucosal membrane is more typical of chronicity (↑↑↑).

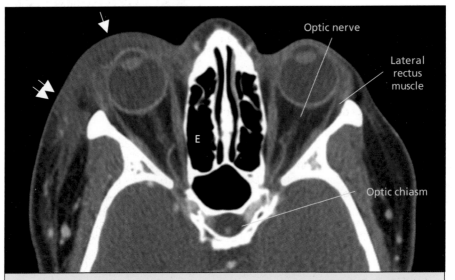

Fig 225 CT scan showing preseptal lid swelling (↑) and periorbital cellulitis (↑↑). The retrobulbar areas of the orbit and the ethmoid (E) sinuses are normal. There are, as yet, normal eye movements and no proptosis. Mild, early cases could be followed up cautiously on an outpatient basis. *Source:* Courtesy of Sandip Basak, MD.

3 Swollen lids (sometimes totally shut); redness and engorgement of conjunctival vessels; clear fluid under conjunctiva (chemosis) (Fig. 226).
4 Loss of eye movement (ophthalmoplegia) due to involvement of CN III, IV, and VI or local damage to extraocular muscles.
5 Rare elevation of intraocular pressure due to venous congestion.

Preseptal cellulitis causes swollen lids which may be totally shut (Figs 217 and 225). This may progress to the rarer and more serious orbital cellulitis (Figs 226 and 227), in which case the globe may not move (ophthalmoplegia) and there is chemosis (conjunctival edema Fig. 293), fever, adenopathy, and exophthalmos. It is due to sinusitis 60% of the time, but also occurs with tooth, facial, or lid infections.

A tough connective tissue called the periorbita lines the inner surface of the orbit.

At the orbital rim, it becomes the orbital septum which then thickens to become the tarsal plate of the lid (see Figs 218 and 178). This continuous fibrous membrane acts as a barrier protecting the orbit from lid and sinus infections and might be considered an "orbital firewall." Beware of the rare breakthrough. If orbital cellulitis occurs, it can easily spread to the cavernous sinus through the superior and inferior ophthalmic veins that drain the orbit and part of the face (Fig. 144). This can cause thrombosis and death. Hospitalize the patient and treat with intravenous antibiotics.

Idiopathic orbital inflammatory syndrome, also known as orbital pseudotumor (Fig. 228), is a non-specific inflammation of the orbit with no identifiable local or systemic cause. It is the third most common orbital disorder behind thyroid and lymphoproliferative disease (see Fig. 229B). An extensive rule-out workup often includes biopsy. Only then may oral, parental, or intralesional steroids be administered.

Exophthalmos

Exophthalmos (proptosis) is a protrusion of the eyeball caused by an increase in orbital contents. It is measured with an exophthalmometer (Fig. 229A). In adults, unilateral and bilateral cases are most often due to thyroid disease (Figs 1-3). In children, unilateral cases are most often due to orbital cellulitis. Other causes are metastatic tumors, orbital hemorrhage, cavernous sinus thrombosis or fistulas, sinus mucoceles,

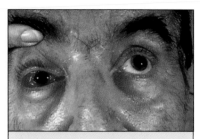

Fig 226 Orbital cellulitis with chemosis and ophthalmoplegia, causing inability to look up.

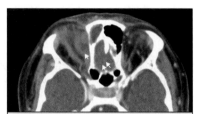

Fig 227 CT scan of orbital cellulitis (↑) caused by ethmoid sinusitis (↑↑). Courtesy of Rand Kirtland, MD.

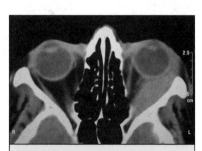

Fig 228 CT scan of left orbital pseudotumor, which is non-infectious inflammation of the orbit. *Source:* Courtesy of Egal Leibovich, MD, and *Arch. Ophthalmol.*, 2007, Vol. 125, No. 12, pp. 1647–1651. Copyright 2007, American Medical Association. All rights reserved.

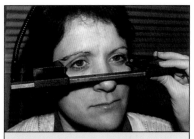

Fig 229A Exophthalmometer.

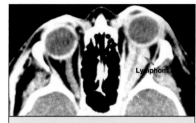

Fig 229B CT scan of orbital lymphoma, exhibiting proptosis.

orbital pseudotumor (Fig. 228), or the following primary orbital tumors:

1 hemangioma
2 rhabdomyosarcoma
3 lipoma
4 dermoid
5 lacrimal gland growth Fig 402–405
6 glioma of the optic nerve
7 lymphoma (Fig. 229B)
8 meningioma (Fig. 124, p. 47)

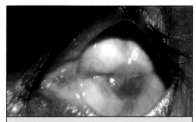

Fig 230 Phthisis bulbi: a shrunken globe. *Source:* Courtesy of University of Iowa, Eyerounds.org.

Enophthalmos

Enophthalmos is a retracted globe. It may be due to loss of orbital fat which is a complication of prostaglandin analogue drugs used to treat glaucoma (Fig. 12). Phthisis bulbi (Fig. 230) is a shrunken globe caused by severe trauma, infection, low pressure, or as a complication of surgery especially for retinal detachments. An eye can incorrectly appear smaller and sunken if the lid droops on that side (Fig. 127) or if the lid on the other eye is elevated (Fig. 177). A blunt blow to the eye can fracture the thin roof of the maxillary sinus (Fig. 231) causing the globe to sink into the orbit. This is called a "blow-out" fracture. Associated signs may include subconjunctival hemorrhage; entrapment of the inferior rectus muscle in the fracture causing restriction of upward gaze; and vertical diplopia (Fig. 232). Decreased sensation (hypesthesia) of the cheek is due to infraorbital nerve damage (Fig. 233). If diplopia or enophthalmos persist, or if more than 50% of the floor is blown out, a silicone, polyethylene, or tita-

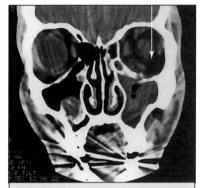

Fig 231 CT scan of an orbital blow-out fracture (↓).

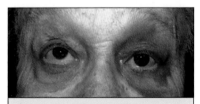

Fig 232 A blow-out fracture may cause entrapment of the inferior rectus muscle resulting in restriction of A upper gaze; lid purpura (hemorrhage).

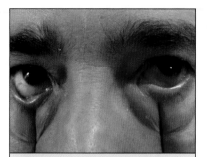

Fig 233 Test for hypesthesia using two paper clips to compare the sensitivity on each side. A positive test indicates injury of the infraorbital nerve (Fig. 108).

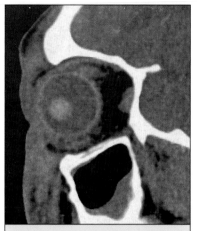

Fig 234 CT scan of traumatic orbital fracture showing lens dislocation.

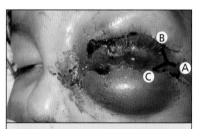

Fig 235 Orbital hemorrhage with overlay of lateral canthal ligament and its superior and inferior branches that connect the tarsal plate to the orbital rim. *Source:* Courtesy of University of Iowa, Eyerounds.org.

nium mesh may be placed under the eye. Any surgery in the orbit should be approached with caution since 1% may result in orbital hemorrhage putting pressure on the optic nerve.

A blow to the eye severe enough to cause a bone fracture could often cause damage to the eyeball. Fig. 234 is a CT scan showing a lens dislocated into the vitreous. Also, be alert to hyphemas, glaucoma, iritis, and retinal detachments.

Orbital hemorrhage is a serious vision threatening emergency (Fig. 235). It is not uncommon for it to occur during orbital surgery or retrobulbar injection of anesthetics, steroids, or antibiotics (Fig. 236). In this closed compartment syndrome, pressure is placed on the optic nerve blood supply. It can be diagnosed by swelling and hemorrhage into the lid and conjunctiva; decreased vision; proptosis of the eye; and elevated eye pressure if it could be measured. It should not be confused with the more common hemorrhage limited to the lid which doesn't threaten vision (Fig. 232). When convinced of the diagnosis—hopefully before 30 minutes—the orbit is decompressed by performing a lateral canthotomy after injecting local anesthetic into the area. Under sterile conditions, a scissor is used to snip the lateral canthal ligament and its two branches (Fig. 235).

Another more common cause of vision threatening compartment syndrome is thyroid orbitopathy in Grave's disease (Figs 1-3).

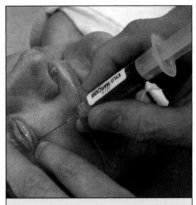

Fig 236 Retrobulbar injections of anesthesia are used for most ocular surgeries to prevent pain and eye movement. Gentle pressure with fingertips for 30 seconds after injection can minimize chance of orbital hemorrhage. In 2020, eye injuries from this injection included globe perforation 60%; retrobulbar hemorrhage 28%; and optic nerve injury 12%. *Source:* Courtesy of University of Iowa, Eyerounds.org.

Chapter 6
Slit lamp examination

The difference between something good and something great is attention to detail.

The slit lamp projects a beam of variable intensity onto the eye, which is viewed through a microscope (Fig. 237). The long, wide beam is useful in scanning surfaces such as lids, conjunctiva, and sclera. The long, narrow beam is for cross-sectional views (Figs 238 and 239). The short, narrow, intense beam is used to study cellular details (Fig. 392).

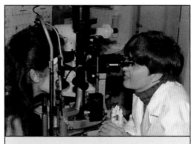

Fig 237 Slit lamp microscope.

Cornea

The cornea is the transparent, anterior continuation of the sclera devoid of both blood and lymphatic vessels. The gray corneoscleral junction is called the limbus. A slit beam cross-section of a normal cornea reveals the following as shown in Figs 240 and 241.

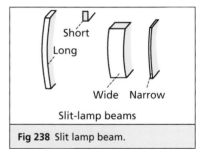

Fig 238 Slit lamp beam.

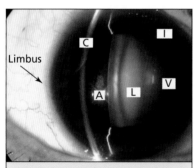

Fig 239 Slit lamp view of anterior segment. C, cornea; A, anterior chamber; I, iris; L, lens; V, vitreous. The limbus, also called the *corneoscleral junction*, has a gray color and is the location of corneal stem cells. It is an important landmark in cataract and retinovitreous surgery. *Source:* Courtesy of Takashi Fujikado, MD.

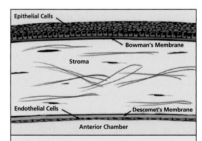

Fig 240 Cross-section of cornea. *Source:* Courtesy of Pfizer Pharmaceuticals. Branches of the sensory trigeminal nerve (CN V) (Fig. 108) enter the stroma from the limbus innervating it and the epithelium. They provide protective and trophic functions. Damage to them (Table 9, p. 94) can cause neurotrophic keratopathy.

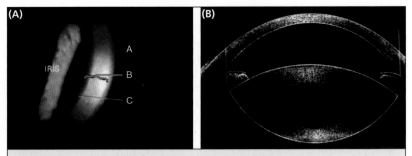

Fig 241 (A) Slit beam cross-section of a cornea. A, epithelium; B, stroma; C, endothelium. (B) Tomogram of anterior segment showing normal thickness of cornea greatest in periphery. *Source:* Courtesy of Richard Witlin, MD.

1 anterior band: epithelium on Bowman's membrane;
2 cross-section: through stroma;
3 posterior band: endothelium on Descemet's membrane.

The corneal epithelium is the superficial covering of the cornea that is four to six layers thick and sits on Bowman's membrane. Its cells regenerate quickly so that 40% of the surface can regenerate in 24 hours. New cells are generated in the deepest layer sitting on Bowman's membrane and move toward the surface under normal conditions. The epithelial cells are also formed from the embryonic stem cells in the limbus (corneoscleral junction) and migrate across the cornea.

The stroma is the clear connective tissue layer and is thinnest in the center of the cornea (545 μm). It is almost twice as thick near the limbus (Fig. 241B). It contains the most densely packed number of sensory fibers in the body, 400 times that of skin. Abrasions and inflammations (keratitis) are, therefore, very painful. "Kerato" is a prefix that refers to cornea.

The deepest endothelial layer sits on Descemet's membrane and is only one cell thick and doesn't regenerate. Its critical function is to pump fluid out of the cornea to maintain clarity.

Corneal epithelial disease

Commonly occurring epithelial abrasions (Figs 242 and 243), due to trauma, present with pain and a "red" eye. Corneal abrasions from playing basketball are the most common sports injury accounting for 17,000 emergency room visits in 2017. The de-epithelialized area stains bright green with fluorescein and a cobalt blue light. Rx: topical antibiotic, a cycloplegic (Cyclogel 1%), and an oral analgesic, with a pressure patch (two patches). Most abrasions clear quickly, within 24–48 hours, largely due to adjacent epithelial cells sliding over the abraded area.

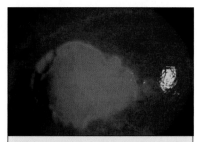

Fig 242 Corneal abrasion stained with fluorescein.

To facilitate the examination of painful eyes, anesthetize with topical proparacaine 0.5%. It acts in seconds and lasts a few minutes. Never prescribe it for relief of pain because continued use damages the cornea.

Rarely, chemical or surgical trauma to the surface is so severe it destroys a large area of the limbus containing epithelial stem cells. In these cases, the epithelium cannot regenerate properly and are replaced by opaque conjunctival epithelium. In this case, a limbal cell transplant has to be done. Normal limbal tissue from the patient's other eye (autograft), from a relative (allograft) (Fig. 244), or from a cadaver may be used.

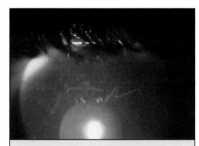

Fig 243 Linear abrasions from trichiasis or particle under lid.

Corneal foreign bodies (FB) (Fig. 245) are removed with a sterile needle after placing two drops of proparacaine anesthetic. Its action begins in 15 seconds and lasts 20 minutes. Do not prescribe for home use since repeated use is toxic. The drop is most commonly used for measurement of eye pressure. The other common location of a particle is under the upper lid. Patients could be advised on the telephone to irrigate the eye at home or grasp the upper lid lashes and pull the lid down and over the lower lid which wipes the undersurface of the lid.

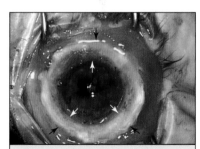

Fig 244 A 360° limbal stem cell allograft: sutured or glued to sclera (↑). *Source:* Courtesy of Clara Chan, MD, and Edward J. Holland, MD, Cincinnati Eye Institute.

Axenfeld nerve loops are intrascleral nerves that commonly appear normally as gray nodules under the bulbar conjunctiva (Fig. 246). Patients with a gritty sensation may confuse

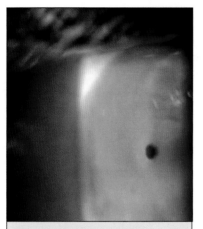

Fig 245 Corneal foreign body. *Source:* Courtesy of University of Iowa, Eyerounds.org.

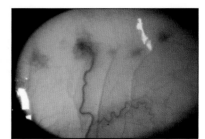

Fig 246 Axenfeld loop. *Source:* Courtesy of University of Iowa, Eyerounds.org.

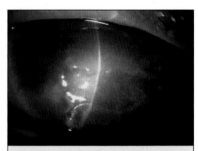

Fig 247 Recurrent corneal erosion with localized epithelial edema.

them with a foreign body and irritate the eyes further by trying to remove.

Localized epithelial edema (Fig. 247, Table 9) has a translucent appearance, unlike an ulcer, which is opaque. In the common condition called recurrent corneal erosion, a small patch of edema develops where the epithelium does not adhere well to Bowman's membrane. This often follows injury, but may be spontaneous.

Table 9 Superficial punctate keratitis (commonly causes photophobia).	
Traumatic causes	*Desiccation*
Contact lenses Ultraviolet light (snow blindness) Entropion causing trichiasis (Fig. 175) Chemical injury Blepharitis Trichiasis (Fig. 234) Rubbing eyes Herpes simplex or zoster Diabetes; LASIK surgery; benzalkonium chloride preservative used in most eye drops.	Dry eye due to decreased tear film production (Fig. 152). Dry eye resulting from increased evaporation due to: 1 inability to close lids after blepharoplasty, 2 Grave's disease (Fig. 1) or lagophthalmos (Fig. 251).

Patients awaken in the morning with pain when cells slough off. This usually occurs just below the center of the cornea. The abrasion is treated with a patch and an antibiotic. The edematous epithelium is treated with hypertonic 2% or 5% sodium chloride solution (Muro 128) in the daytime and sodium chloride 5% ophthalmic ointment (Muro 128 ointment) at bedtime. If sloughing continues, roughing up Bowman's membrane with a needle (stromal puncture) increases adhesiveness of cells.

Superficial punctate keratitis (SPK) (Figs 248 and 249, Fig. 9) is epithelial edema, which appears as punctate hazy areas that stain with fluorescein. Burning, pain, conjunctival redness, and blurry vision may result, which is most common with dry eye. Inferior corneal edema occurs with an inability to close the lids, as occurs in Bell's palsy (Figs 111 and 112), Grave's disease (Fig. 1), lagophthalmos (Fig. 251), and with blepharitis of lower lid due to local release of toxic secretions. Loss of corneal nerves could occur from diabetes and following LASIK surgery and could result in dry eye with epithelial edema. The reduced corneal sensation following LASIK surgery and in diabetes (neurotrophic keratitis) may also cause dry eye and epithelial edema. Human fetal amniotic membrane may be used to reduce inflammation and speed epithelial healing. It is placed on the cornea when healing is not occurring. It lasts 2–10 days (Prokera or Ambiodisc).

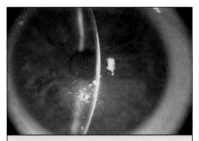

Fig 248 Superficial punctate keratitis (SPK) see Table 9, p. 94.

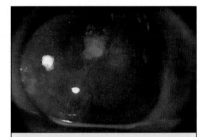

Fig 249 SPK stained with fluorescein.

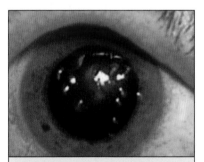

Fig 250 Filamentary keratitis presents with strings of epithelium and is often due to dry eye. *Source:* Courtesy of University of Iowa, Eyerounds.org.

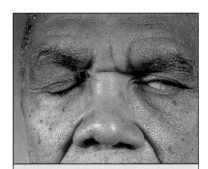

Fig 251 Lagophthalmos is a condition in which the lids don't close completely. This commonly occurs from facial nerve paralysis in Bell's palsy.

Table 10 Conjunctivitis - redness more pronounced in peripheral conjunctiva (see Figs 305 and 395).

	Viral	Bacterial	Allergic
Onset	Acute	Acute	Intermittent
Associated complaints	Often sore throat, rhinitis, fever	Often none	History of allergy; nasal or sinus stuffiness, dermatitis
Discharge	Watery	Thick, yellow	Stringy mucus
Preauricular node	Common	Infrequent	None

Filamentary keratitis is an irritating, light-sensitizing overgrowth of degenerated corneal epithelial cells. The strands of cells are often multiple and most often due to aging, dry eye, and trauma. They may be removed with a Nd:YAG laser (Fig. 250), but may recur. Prevent by treating underlying cause.

Corneal vascularization is a response to injury. Superficial vessels are most commonly a response to poorly fitting contact lenses (Figs 253 and 255), but also grow into areas damaged from ulcers, lacerations, or chemicals.

Chemical injuries with basic chemicals such as lye are most ominous because they immediately penetrate the depths of the cornea and permanently scar (Figs 254 and 255). Acid burns usually do not penetrate the stroma or scar. Rx: irrigate all chemical injuries immediately and profusely.

Epidemic keratoconjunctivitis (Fig. 256) is a common, highly infectious condition due to one of the adenoviruses that cause the common cold. There may be a severe conjunctivitis lasting up to 3 weeks associated with photophobia, fever, cold symptoms, and an adenopathy. The main problem is the keratitis, which can last for months or, rarely, years. It rarely scars, but does restrict use of contact lenses until it clears. Wash your hands, instruments, chair, and doorknobs especially well after evaluating this eye infection. Diluted povidone-iodine appears effective against virus in tears, but not replicating virus in cells.

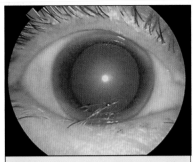

Fig 252 SPK from trichiasis.

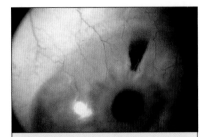

Fig 253 Superficial vascularization, often due to poorly fitting contact lenses. *Source:* Courtesy of Michael Kelly.

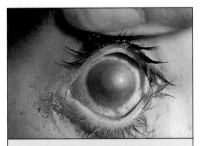

Fig 254 Sodium hydroxide injury minutes after the event.

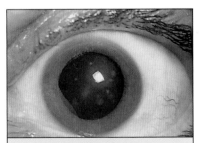

Fig 256 Epidemic keratoconjunctivitis with characteristic white, punctate subepithelial infiltrates.

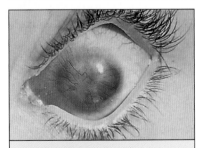

Fig 255 Sodium hydroxide injury months after the event.

It may be placed topically in office and rinsed out in 2 minutes. Topical steroid may relieve symptoms but could prolong the course. Unlike most other viruses, this adenovirus can be hardy, and may be cultured from dry surfaces for weeks.

Herpes simplex virus type 1 (HSV-1) is very common on the face, especially around the eyes and lips and is often triggered by stress. At age 4, about 25% of the population is seropositive, and this approaches 100% by age 60. When the corneal epithelium (Figs 257 and 258) is involved, the lesions, called *dendrites*, appear and are similar in appearance to a branching tree, especially when stained with fluorescein. Diffuse punctate or round lesions can also occur and mimic the lesions due to dry eye and blepharitis. Patients complain of a gritty ocular sensation, conjunctivitis, and a history of a fever sore on the lip, nose, or mouth. Herpes often decreases corneal sensation. This can be tested by comparing sensation in eye by touching both with a cotton-tipped applicator, obviously testing the uninfected eye first. There may be small vesicles on the skin of the lids (Fig. 260), which often crust and then disappear within 3 weeks. Involvement of the surface epithelium of the cornea rarely causes scarring and loss of vision unlike the deeper stromal keratitis and uveitis. When the virus involvement does penetrate into the stroma (Fig. 259), cautious

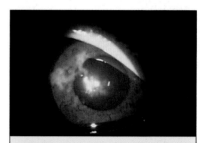

Fig 257 Herpes simplex keratitis with tree-like branching lesions.

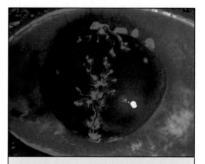

Fig 258 Herpes simplex with large fluorescein-stained dendrites. Lesions may also be patchy. Confusion could occur with smaller staining punctate dots which are more often due to dry eye, blepharitis, contact lenses, other viruses, or drug toxicity (Figs 252 and 256). *Source:* Courtesy of Allan Connor, Princess Margaret Hospital, Toronto, Canada.

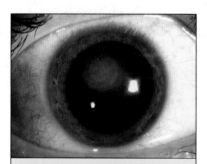

Fig 259 Herpetic inflammation of the stroma could cause permanent scarring with loss of vision. Therefore, steroid eyedrops may be cautiously added. *Source:* Courtesy of University of Iowa, Eyerounds, org.

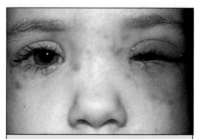

Fig 260 Herpes dermatitis with multiple small blisters.

addition of topical corticosteroids, together with antivirals, may minimize this scarring and the resulting decrease in vision. This permanent structural change of the stroma, causing haze and loss of vision, when severe, accounts for three percent of all penetrating corneal transplants done in the USA. Recurrences are common. Rx: Generic trifluridine (Viroptic) 1% every 2 hours has been the mainstay treatment for years, but branded Zirgan gel, ganciclovir 0.15%, can be used every 3 hours and is less toxic. Both are usually used during waking hours. Acyclovir 500 mg PO BID may be added in resistant cases, or for systemic symptoms.

Anxious patients must be reassured that this HSV-1 condition, causing corneal disease, is not usually due to HSV-2, which is a venereal disease transmitted by sexual contact, although HSV-2 can, less often, spread to the cornea.

Corneal ulcers are usually caused by a bacterial infection, although they may occasionally be the result of a viral, parasitic, or fungal infection. They are characterized by conjunctivitis with pain and white corneal infiltrates. Over 50% result from contact lens wear, especially lenses worn during sleep. Other causes often include corneal abrasions, conjunctivitis, and blepharitis. Treat vigorously on an emergency basis, since it almost always scars and, in the case of *Pseudomonas*, may perforate within 1 day (Figs 261–263). Treatment often consists of more than one antibiotic drop and ointment (see Table 8, p.70). The initial frequency of instillation may be as often as every 15 minutes through the night when the central visual axis is involved.

Marginal ulcers (Fig. 261) are most common and may be due to infection or an immune reaction to staphylococcus toxins from associated chronic blepharitis. Rx: topical hourly broad-spectrum antibiotics (Table 8). Steroids are sometimes used to suppress the inflammation from staphylococcal toxins and when a herpetic cause is confidently ruled out. Treat the often present blepharitis with lid scrubs, warm compresses, and massage of the lid margin.

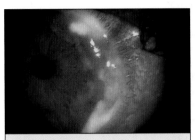
Fig 261 Marginal corneal ulcer.

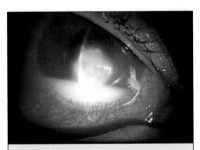
Fig 262 Central corneal ulcer with secondary hypopyon.

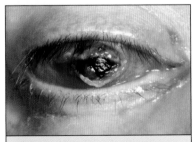
Fig 263 Perforated corneal ulcer. *Source:* Courtesy of Elliot Davidoff, MD.

Central ulcers (Fig. 262) are most ominous and, in such cases, cultures are always needed. Multiple topical broad-spectrum antibiotics are used up to every 15 minutes. The infection infrequently enters the globe (Fig. 262). When it does, a level of white cells may be seen in the anterior chamber, which is the space bounded anteriorly by the cornea and posteriorly by the iris and lens. This is called a *hypopyon* (Figs 262 and 456) and might require a culture of the interior eye, especially if the vitreous is also involved. When ulcers show no positive cultures for bacteria and are nonresponsive to multiple broad-spectrum antibiotics, one must next consider viral infections, most commonly herpes simplex or parasites and fungus. Acanthamoeba is a parasite that commonly occurs in fresh water. It uncommonly causes ulcers in contact lens wearers, especially from dirty cases and also from swimming in contaminated water. Fungal infections may cause 3% of corneal ulcers in temperate zones and up to 35% in the tropics. The incidence increases from overuse of topical antibacterials and steroids when treating keratitis and also from injuries from plant material such as a branch or thorn.

Corneal endothelial disease

A monolayer of endothelial cells covers the deepest layer of the cornea and pumps fluid from the stroma to maintain corneal clarity. There are usually 2800 endothelial cells/mm², and they do not replicate. When the number of cells drops below 500, or cells are damaged, corneal edema can occur, causing blurry vision and discomfort (Figs 264–266). The most common cause for this edema is cataract surgery. In these cases, the endothelial cells may be injured mechanically, chemically, or from rejection of the lens implant. This complication of cataract surgery is the most common reason leading to the need for corneal transplant surgery. Extremely elevated eye pressure (over 35 mmHg; Figs 364 and 371), iritis, and a genetic weakness of the endothelium in Fuchs' dystrophy (Figs 268 and 269) are also common causes. Very high pressure,

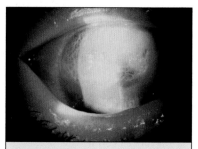

Fig 264 Severe corneal edema with epithelial cysts is referred to as *bullous keratopathy*. It reduces vision and is usually very uncomfortable, often breaking down to painful corneal abrasions. *Source:* Courtesy of Kenneth R. Kenyon, MD, and *Arch. Ophthalmol.*, Mar. 1976, Vol. 94, pp. 494–495. Copyright 1976, American Medical Association. All rights reserved.

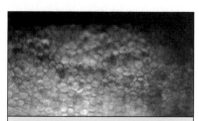

Fig 265 At birth, the normal endothelial cell count is 5,000 cells/mm. It steadily decreases with age. Shown here is specular microscopy scan of normal endothelial cell count, 2800 cells/mm² at 60 years of age.

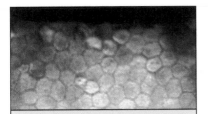

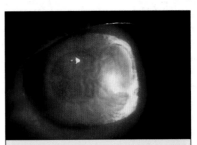

Fig 266 Specular microscopy after cataract surgery that damaged the endothelium and caused corneal edema, resulting in a cell count of 680 cells/mm². If cells are damaged, they do not multiply to fill the gap. Instead, they enlarge and lose their normal hexagonal shape and their ability to pump fluid from the cornea. *Source:* Courtesy of Martin Schneider, MD.

Fig 267 Edematous folds in the cornea – called stria – usually result from low intraocular pressure. It is a similar effect to a balloon not fully blown up.

often over 40 mmHg in acute-angle glaucoma, temporarily damages the endothelium causing corneal edema with the classic symptom of halos around lights. Symmetrel (amantadine), used to treat Parkinson's disease, could cause corneal edema by decreasing the endothelial cell count. Low pressure, below 5 mmHg, could also cause corneal cloudiness with stria (Fig. 267).

Fuchs' dystrophy is a genetic disorder of the Descemet's endothelial complex (Figs 268 and 269) that leads to a drop in endothelial cells. It occurs in 5% of the US population. It is

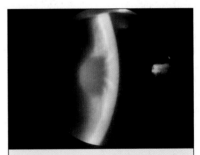

Fig 268 Fuchs' dystrophy with central corneal thickening and haze due to edema. *Source:* Courtesy of Hank Perry, MD.

Healthy	Pleomorphism	Polymegatism	Guttata

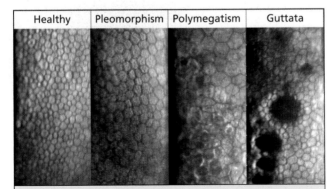

Fig 269 Endothelial cell changes in aging with guttata due to Fuch's dystrophy. *Source:* Courtesy of Jorge E. Valdez-Garcia and Jorge L. Domeno Hickman, Institute do Oftalmologia Technologico de Monterrey.

bilateral and identified by guttata, which are small, round spots of thickening in Descemet's membrane. They are usually in the central corneal axis. It could lead to corneal edema and eventually require corneal endothelial cell transplant surgery (Fig. 270).

Corneal transplantation (keratoplasty)

Keratoplasty is one of the most successful organ transplant surgeries with more than a 90% success rate at 1 year and 80% after 10 years. In 2019, 46,500 procedures were performed in the USA using donor corneas from eye banks. The FDA approved storage of donor corneas up to 14 days but most surgeons prefer a fresher 3–7 day specimen. Unlike other transplant surgeries, like kidney and heart, there is almost no wait for donor corneas. More than one-third of donor corneas are rejected by US eye banks if the donors died having infections, certain cancers, and Parkinson's or Alzheimer's disease. Penetrating keratoplasty (Figs 270 and 271)—a full-thickness technique—is used to replace scarred, opacified stroma. Problems with penetrating keratoplasty are that it requires extensive suturing, which remains in place for over a year. It could take that amount of time for vision to return. Also, there is often a lot of residual astigmatism. If the stroma is clear, and the only pathology is in the endothelium, an endothelial keratoplasty (DSEK) Figs 272–276) may be performed. In 2019, 17,409 penetrating, and 30,650 endothelial replacement keratoplasties were performed in the USA. Over 10,000 were done in 2019.

A third type of keratoplasty, called deep anterior lamellar keratoplasty (DALK), is done less frequently (1000 procedures/year) for eyes with stromal opacities and healthy endothelium (Figs 277–281). In DALK, just the anterior cornea is replaced, leaving behind a significant amount of posterior stroma with the endothelium and Descemet's membrane. Its advantage is that it can remove anterior

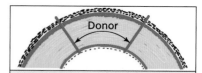

Fig 270 Diagram outlining full-thickness corneal transplant (penetrating keratoplasty).

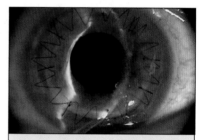

Fig 271 Full-thickness corneal transplant (penetrating keratoplasty).

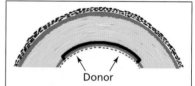

Fig 272 Descemet-stripping endothelial keratoplasty (DSEK): After removing damaged endothelium and Descemet's membrane, the donor tissue is folded to fit through a small wound. Unscrolling the implant is the most difficult step. An air bubble is injected to press the donor graft against the cornea. The endothelial cells' natural pumping action holds the graft in place without sutures (Fig. 275).

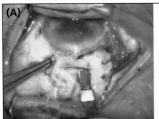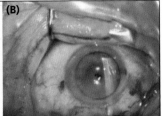

Fig 273 Replacement of endothelium and Descemet's membrane. (A) Stripping of an 8.0 mm diameter of diseased endothelium and Descemet's membrane. (B) Insertion of folded donor graft. *Source:* Studeny Pavel, Farkis A. et al., *Br. J. Ophthalmol.*, 2010, Vol. 94, No. 7. Reproduced with permission of BMJ Publishing Group, Ltd.

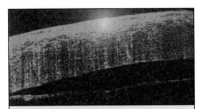

Fig 274 OCT showing detached endothelial graft. *Source:* Courtesy of Amar Agarwal, MD.

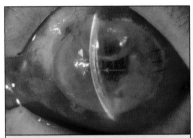

Fig 275 DSEK graft separation (↑) 3 days after transplant. It was reattached by injecting an air bubble. *Source:* Courtesy of Christopher Rapuano, MD, Wills Eye Hospital.

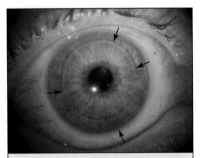

Fig 276 Successful DSEK surgery with 8.0 mm implant in place (↑). *Source:* Courtesy of Henry Perry, MD.

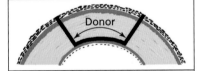

Fig 277 DALK removes most of the stroma up to Descemet's membrane. A common complication is damage to the remaining thin, 10 μm layer. This complication necessitates converting to a penetrating keratoplasty 20% of the time.

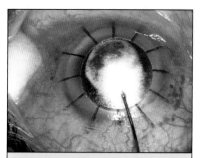

Fig 278 DALK: step 1 is to inject air into the corneal stroma to begin separation of stroma from Descemet's membrane. It is a difficult step in avoiding perforation of Descemet's membrane.

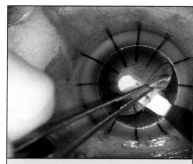

Fig 279 DALK: step 2 is to complete stromal dissection with crescent blade.

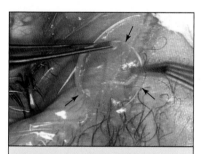

Fig 280 DALK: step 3 is to remove Descemet's membrane from donor cornea (↑).

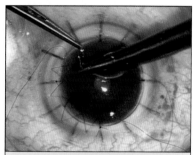

Fig 281 DALK: step 4 is to suture donor graft to recipient bed. *Source*: D.C.Y. Han et al., *Am. J. Ophthalmol.*, 2009, Vol. 148, No. 5, pp. 744–751. Reproduced permission of Elsevier.

corneal opacities, leaving behind the patient's own endothelial cells. Immunologic rejection of donor endothelial cells is the leading cause of full thickness corneal graft failure.

A human corneal donor graft may be repeatedly rejected for immune reasons or because of a poor surface environment, as with dry eye or with a vascularized cornea that occurs with chemical burns (Figs 254 and 255). A last effort at maintaining clarity in the central axis is implantation of a graft utilizing a centrally located plastic lens. In 2007, 639 grafts of the Boston type were performed (Figs 282 and 283). Retroprosthetic membranes and glaucoma are more common complications, especially in children.

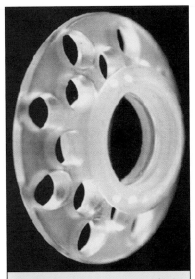

Fig 282 The Boston Keratoprosthesis: collar-button device made of PMMA plastic. It is incorporated into a corneal graft that serves as a carrier sutured in place like a standard graft.

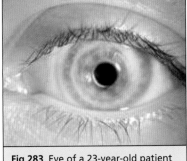

Fig 283 Eye of a 23-year-old patient with congenital endothelial dystrophy. Four standard corneal grafts had failed. A Boston Keratoprosthesis implanted 5 years earlier resulted in consistent vision of 20/30 and normal pressure. *Source*: Courtesy of Claes Dohlman, MD, PhD.

Keratoconus (Figs 284–287) is a bilateral central thinning and bulging (ectasia) of the cornea to a conical shape with possible scarring. It is due to weakening of the stromal collagen. There may be an orange epithelial deposition of iron around the base of the cone called Fleischer's ring. It begins between ages 10 and 30, often in allergic persons. Rubbing the eye may cause or worsen the condition and should be discouraged. Once keratoconus is identified, topical anti-allergic medications and lubricants should be prescribed to eliminate rubbing. There is a higher incidence within families.

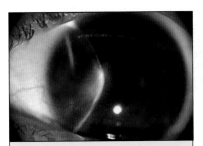

Fig 284 Keratoconus with scarring at apex of cone.

The resulting irregular type of astigmatism corrects poorly with glasses and may need soft or gas-permeable contact lenses to obtain clearer vision.

If the cornea continues to steepen, one may flatten and strengthen it with intracorneal rings (Fig. 286) or more often chemically strengthening the stromal collagen using a technique called corneal cross-linking. In this

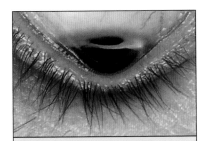

Fig 285 Munson's sign: conical cornea indents lid when looking down. *Source*: Courtesy of Michael P. Kelly.

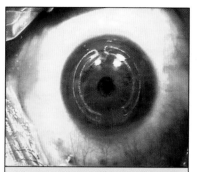

Fig 286 Intracorneal ring strengthens and flattens the cornea in keratoconus and is a less used alternative to chemical cross-linking. One advantage is that it may reduce myopia and astigmatism. Rarely, ring migration could cause corneal melting. *Source*: Courtesy of Dimitri Azar, MD.

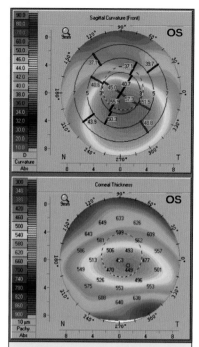

Fig 287 Corneal tomography of keratoconus showing thin, steep, eccentrically located corneal apex having a 57.3 D power with a thickness of only 449 μm. Normal central cornea averages 43 D with a thickness of 545 μm. Also diagnostic of keratoconus is a posterior corneal surface that is steeper (conical) than the anterior surface. *Source*: Courtesy of Richard Witlin, MD.

procedure, most surgeons have the best results by first removing the corneal epithelium. Then, riboflavin 0.1% solution is continuously dropped onto the cornea while the eye is irradiated with UVA light for 30 minutes. It should only be used in cases of documented progression of disease. It may be used to slow or even halt progression. Severe keratoconus is treated with penetrating keratoplasty and accounts for 20% of corneal transplantation in the USA.

Down's syndrome occurs in about 1 in 5000 births and is due to trisomy of chromosome 21. It is characterized by mental retardation, short stature, and a transverse palmar crease ("simian crease"). There is an increased incidence of keratoconus, strabismus, cataracts, and refractive errors (Fig. 288).

Argyrosis results from long-term exposure to topical or systemic silver (Fig. 289). Silver nitrate 2% eye drops were used extensively as an anti-infective in the first half of the twentieth century. It was the mainstay prophylactic therapy in newborns. Before its discovery in 1881 by Carl Crede, 1 in 300 newborns were blinded by ophthalmia neonatorium. Erythromycin ointment has now replaced it in the delivery room as a routine prophylactic.

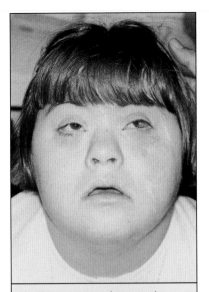

Fig 288 Down's syndrome patient with keratoconus. Corneal edema (hydrops) is caused by a tear in Descemet's membrane. Also, note the characteristic flat face, small nose, low nasal bridge, narrow interpupillary distance, and upward slanting palpebral fissures. *Source*: Courtesy of Kenneth R. Kenyon, MD, and *Arch. Ophthalmol.*, Mar. 1976, Vol. 94, pp. 494–495, Copyright 1976, American Medical Association., All rights reserved.

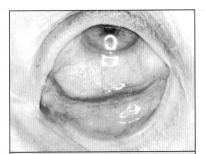

Fig 289 Argyrosis: deposition of silver in conjunctiva, cornea, and lid. Silver nitrate eye drops were universally instilled in the eyes of newborns in the hospital nursery, but the practice has replaced by using broad-spectrum antibiotic drops or ointments. *Source*: Courtesy of Elliott Davidoff, MD.

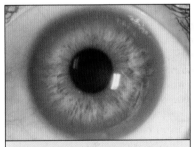

Fig 290 Copper deposited in Descemet's membrane causing an orange ring at the limbus (Kayser–Fleischer ring) pathognomonic of Wilson's disease. Compare with corneal arcus shown in Appendix 1 (Fig. 589). *Source*: Courtesy of Denise de Freitas, MD. Paulista School of Medicine, Sao Paulo, Brazil.

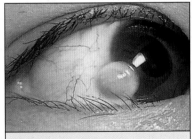

Fig 291 Corneal dermoid.

Wilson's disease (hepatolenticular degeneration) is characterized by excessive deposition of copper in the liver and brain. It is a rare autosomal recessive disorder that often begins before age 40. The plasma copper-carrying protein – serum ceruloplasmin – is low. The pathognomonic sign of the condition is the brownish or gray-green Kayser– Fleischer ring (Fig. 290) due to copper deposits in Descemet's membrane, adjacent to the limbus.

Dermoid tumors (Fig. 291) are benign congenital growths often having protruding hairs. They are most common at the corneal limbus or in the orbit and may grow during puberty. They are removed if vision is threatened, or for discomfort and cosmetic reasons.

Conjunctiva

The conjunctiva is a mucous membrane. The bulbar conjunctiva covers the sclera and ends at the corneal limbus. The palpebral conjunctiva lines the lids (Fig. 292). Fluid within the conjunctiva is called *chemosis* (Fig. 293) and is commonly seen in allergy, but also in infectious conjunctivitis, Grave's disease, and in rare cases of orbital venous congestion.

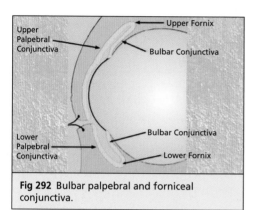

Fig 292 Bulbar palpebral and forniceal conjunctiva.

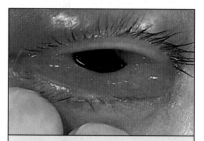

Fig 293 Chemosis refers to conjunctival edema.

To examine the inner surface of the upper lid or to massage the meibomian glands in the case of blepharitis, first warn the patient, then "flip the lid" as follows:

1 have the patient look down with eyes open,
2 grasp eyelashes of upper lid at their bases,
3 pull out and up on lashes while pushing in and down on upper tarsal margin (patient should continue to look down during examination),
4 to return lid to normal position, have the patient look up.

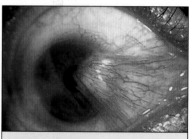

Fig 294 Pterygium.

A pterygium (Fig. 294) is a triangular growth of vascularized conjunctiva encroaching on the nasal cornea. Two causes are wind and ultraviolet light. It may be excised for cosmetic, comfort, or visual reasons. Recurrences of up to 30–40% are reported, but are significantly reduced to 2% by replacing excised conjunctiva with an autograft (Figs 295 and 296).

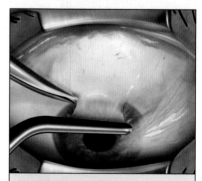

Fig 295 Excision of conjunctival autograft which is usually harvested from the superior bulbar conjunctiva.

A pinguecula (Figs 297 and 298) is a common, benign, yellowish elevation of the 180° conjunctiva, usually nasal, but also temporal. It is composed of collagen and elastic tissue, and occasionally becomes red, especially with allergies, sunlight, and dust. It is infrequently removed at the slit lamp if it is chronically inflamed; if it interferes with contact lens wear; or if it is a cosmetic problem.

Subconjunctival hemorrhages (Fig. 299) may be spontaneous. Common causes include rubbing of the eye or Valsalva maneuvers, as occurs with coughing, sneezing, constipation, and heavy lifting. Elevated blood pressure and anticoagulants may increase the incidence.

Lymphangiectasia refers to the engorgement of conjunctival lymphatic channels, most notably on the bulbar conjunctiva (Fig. 300). It is usually benign with no apparent cause, but may be related to allergy. When symptomatic, it may be cauterized or excised.

Conjunctival concretions are commonly occurring, often multiple, small, benign, hard yellowish-white deposits of inspissated

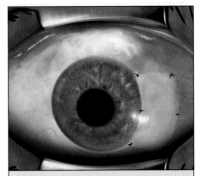

Fig 296 Autograft is usually sutured (rarely glued) to nasal bulbar conjunctiva after removal of pterygium.

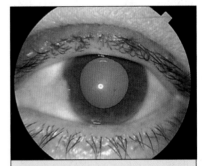

Fig 297 A pinguecula is a very common benign yellow elevation of the conjunctiva most often at the nasal limbus.

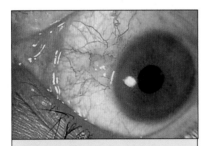

Fig 298 Pingueculitis.

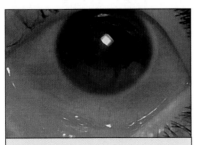

Fig 299 Subconjunctival hemorrhage.

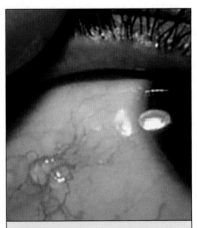

Fig 300 Lymphangiectasia. *Source*: Courtesy of University of Iowa, Eyerounds.org.

degenerative matter buried under the superficial palpebral conjunctiva (Fig. 301). They are usually asymptomatic unless the overlying conjunctiva erodes, at which time they cause a gritty sensation. Unexplained surface irritation especially with corneal fluorescein staining mandates examination under the upper lid. They may be removed at the slit lamp using a topical anesthetic and sterile needle.

Conjunctival verruca (papilloma) is a benign growth initiated after infection by human papillomavirus (Fig. 302) and more often appears on the skin (Fig. 187). A symblepharon (Figs 10 and 304) is an adhesion of the bulbar and palpebral conjunctiva. Contracture can lead to an entropion with trichiasis. It is most commonly due to chemical burns, trachoma, epidemic keratoconjunctivitis, and two of the following immune blistering mucocutaneous diseases.

1 Stevens–Johnson syndrome is an acute blistering immune reaction to a foreign antigen, usually a drug (Fig. 10). It can affect the skin and/or the eyes and could be fatal.
2 Pemphigoid (Fig. 303) is a rare autoimmune condition causing fluid-filled blisters involving the skin and conjunctiva. It could last for years, and unlike Stevens–Johnson, it is not fatal. It is also confirmed by biopsy. *Pemphix* is Latin for "blister."

Conjunctivitis, (inflammation of the conjunctiva, see Table 10, p. 96) causes redness with a gritty sensation. Common causes are tired eyes, pollutants, wind, dust, allergy, or

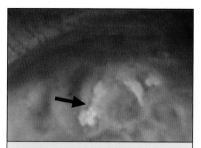

Fig 301 Conjunctival concretions. *Source*: Courtesy of University of Iowa, Eyerounds.org.

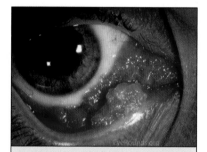

Fig 302 Conjunctival verruca (wart) with typical cauliflower appearance. *Source:* Courtesy of University of Iowa, Eyerounds.org.

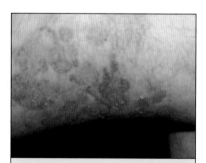

Fig 303 Pemphigoid causes itchy, red blisters on the skin and conjunctiva

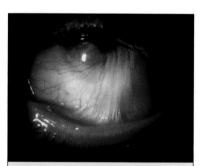

Fig 304 Symblepharon: adhesions of bulbar to palpebral conjunctiva should be lysed with a glass rod or wet cotton applicator to prevent permanent scar. *Source*: Kheirkhah et al., *Am. J. Ophthalmol.*, 2008, Vol. 146, p. 271. Reproduced with permission of Elsevier.

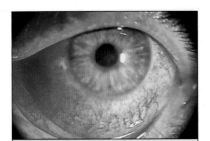

Fig 305 Conjunctivitis is usually due to a bacterial or viral infection. Allergy causes less redness.

infection (Fig. 305). If there is pain, it usually indicates corneal or intraocular involvement. Vascularized elevations of the palpebral conjunctiva, called papillae (Fig. 306), are most characteristic of giant papillary conjunctivitis and vernal conjunctivitis.

Giant papillary conjunctivitis (or GPC) is a common cause for rejecting soft contact lenses. Large papillae develop under the lids. They are an immune reaction, usually in response to mucous debris on the lenses, and are more common in allergic individuals. Rx: change to a contact lens that is disposed of more frequently, i.e., every 2 weeks or even on a daily schedule; decrease wearing time; keep lenses especially clean; and sometimes discontinue lens wear.

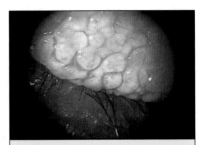

Fig 306 Papillae of the palpebral conjunctiva.

Vernal keratoconjunctivitis is an allergic condition in which large papillae are under the upper lid. They could abrade the cornea. It occurs in the first decade and may last for years. Both giant papillary conjunctivitis and vernal conjunctivitis may be treated with a topical mast cell inhibitor such as Cromolyn 4% solution. Sometimes steroid drops are also needed.

White lymphoid elevations of the conjunctiva (Fig. 307), called follicles, occur as a reaction to conjunctival irritation, especially from viruses, *Chlamydia*, and drugs.

1 Trachoma is a severe keratoconjunctivitis due to an infection by *Chlamydia trachomatis*. The worldwide risk has been reduced from 1–5 billion in 2002 to 142 million in 2019 due to mass treatment with antibiotics, improved

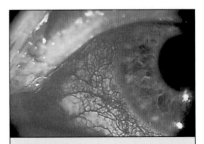

Fig 307 Follicles of the palpebral conjunctiva.

facial cleanliness, and access to clean water and sanitation. It is responsible for blindness in 6 million people outside the USA. It begins with papillae and follicles on the superior palpebral conjunctiva. Conjunctival shortening may result in an entropion, which causes trichiasis. Inflammation of the cornea leads to superior vascularization (pannus), occasional corneal scarring, and loss of vision (Figs 306–308). Rx: a single dose of azithromycin, 20 mg/kg.

2 Inclusion conjunctivitis in adults is a follicular conjunctivitis (Fig. 307) with occasional keratitis. It is also due to *Chlamydia trachomatis* of a different serotype than that causing trachoma. This organism is the most common sexually transmitted pathogen and is the primary notifiable disease to the US Centers for Disease Control and Prevention. The number of reported cases of treatable sexually transmitted diseases in the USA has increased for the past three years with the latest number of cases of chlamydia, 1.8 million; syphilis, 115,045; and gonorrhea, 820,000. Newborns had 1.306 cases of syphilis (Figs 414 and 415); 900,000 cases of chlamydia; and 200,000 cases of gonorrhea. Within hours after birth, erythromycin ointment, or a choice of antibiotic eye drops which may include Vigamox, Tobrex, or Ciprofloxin (Table 8, p. 70); or less often, silver nitrate (Fig. 289).

Bacterial conjunctivitis has a white-yellow discharge and is often due to *Staphylococcus aureus*, *Streptococcus pneumonia*, and *Haemophilus influenzae*. It is usually treated without cultures (Figs 309 and 310) with inexpensive generic medications (see Table 8, p. 70). Ointments blur vision and are most useful for bedtime use. Blepharitis (Figs 153, 154, 206–216, and 310) should be suspected in cases of chronic recurring conjunctivitis, sties, and chalazia.

Viruses cause half the cases of infectious conjunctivitis (Figs 309, 310, 395, Tables 8, p.70 and 10, p. 96). They are more often bilateral with profuse tearing and are usually associated with "cold symptoms" and swollen preauricular and submandibular nodes (Fig. 148). Viral

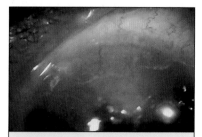

Fig 308 Corneal inflammation from trachoma.

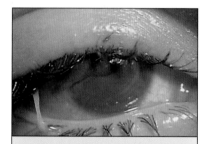

Fig 309 Infectious conjunctivitis: Assume conjunctivitis – "pink eye" – of any type, has an infectious discharge and tear film. Wash your hands and instruments thoroughly and remind patients to do the same and use their own towels. Epidemic keratoconjunctivitis (Fig. 256) is especially contagious, and office doorknobs should be cleansed. AIDS virus was only found in bloody tears, but treat cautiously. Only 1 in 30 COVID-19 patients with severe respiratory symptoms had the virus in their tears, and it was only in the one patient that had conjunctivitis.

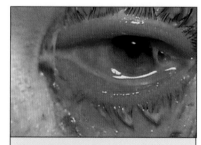

Fig 310 Bacterial blepharoconjunctivitis.

causes are more likely when the condition doesn't respond to topical antibiotics (Table 8, p. 70). Cultures are not usually practical. Antibiotic/steroid combinations may relieve symptoms, but could aggravate an atypical herpes simplex infection which can be ruled out with a slit lamp exam.

Allergic conjunctivitis is a condition associated with intermittent itching, minimal conjunctival injection, stringy mucous discharge, chemosis, and puffy lids. Conjunctival injection aggravated by exposure to airborne allergens, U-V light, or dry air is sometimes limited to exposed conjunctiva in palpebral fissure. It is revealed by spreading the lids apart and seeing white conjunctiva under the covered lids. Treatment begins with avoidance of known irritants, discontinuing makeup and applying cold compresses. When drops are needed, begin with over-the-counter drugs and then generic prescriptions, since they are less expensive and very effective. First line drops, when needed, may have combinations of the following three ingredients: decongestants, antihistamines, or mast cell inhibitors. Naphazoline "decongestant," combined with an antihistamine "pheniramine" is sold under the brand names Opcon A, Visine A, and Naphcon A. That decongestant with the antihistamine antazoline is called Albalon A. Two problems with these adrenergic decongestants that "get the red out" is that it may cause a rebound redness when discontinued. Also, they dilate the pupil and infrequently may cause narrow angle glaucoma (Figs 363 and 364).

So ask patient to call if they have the rare onset of sudden pain and redness.

Mast cells, found in connective tissue throughout the body are part of the immune system and contain histamine granules. Examples of commonly recommended mast cell stabilizing drops are generic, once a day, olepatadine (Pataday); generic, twice a day, azelastine (Optivar); cromolyn (Crolom); or natatifin (Alaway, Zaditor). Mast cell inhibitors may be preferred for more chronic use in more difficult-to-treat cases. A second line drop is the non-steroidal anti-inflammatory drug (NSAID) ketorolac (Acular), which may be used up to q.i.d. It reduces the release of prostaglandin (see Table 14, p. 145) that causes inflammation. The third go-to therapy include steroid drugs, which may be used by themselves or added to the prior two groups. Because of more side effects, including increased eye pressure and reduced immunity to infection, especially herpes simplex, it is usually prescribed with the guidance of an eye care professional. Steroids with the least side effects are fluorometholone (FML) or loteprednol (Alrex). Dosage is adjusted to control symptoms. Minor eye irritations causing redness could be treated with over-the-counter brimonidine 0.025% (Lumify) which acts in minutes and lasts up to eight hours.

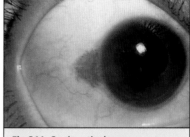

Fig 311 Conjunctival nevus.

Oral antihistamines may be added. "Allergy shots" (immunotherapy) are usually reserved for more severe, chronic cases. After skin testing for sensitivity, an allergist may inject small amounts of the offending allergen over a 3–5-year period.

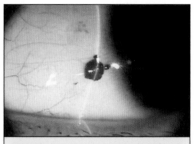

Fig 312 Conjunctival melanoma.

Conjunctival nevi (Fig. 311), often brown in color, are common. Malignant transformation of nevi to melanomas is rare. Malignant transformation is suggested by satellites, rapid growth, elevation, and inflammation (Fig. 312) and occurs 75% of the time from a pre-existing benign pigmented lesion.

Ocular melanosis oculi refers to hyperpigmentation of ocular structures including the iris, the choroid, and the trabecular meshwork, the latter of which may cause glaucoma. The episclera and sclera may appear slate blue (Fig. 313). When the skin is involved it is called oculodermal melanocytosis (nevus of Ota). This condition is associated with a high rate of melanoma and should be monitored (Figs 380–387).

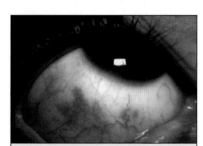

Fig 313 Melanosis oculi with cutaneous involvement (lower right) has a 4× increased chance of developing a uveal melanoma. *Source*: Courtesy of University of Iowa, Eyerounds.org.

Sclera

The sclera is the white, fibrous, protective outer coating of the eye that is continuous with the cornea. The episclera is a thin layer of vascularized tissue that covers the sclera. Its venous network drains the aqueous from Schlemm's canal and the uveoscleral pathway (Figs 319–322). Obstruction anywhere in this system causes high eye pressure resulting in glaucoma. The main glaucoma medications (prostaglandin-analogues) lower eye pressure by opening this uveoscleral pathway leading to the episcleral veins (Fig. 321).

Tenon's capsule is a thin, fibrous membrane lying between the sclera and conjunctiva. Subtenon's injections of drugs, most commonly steroids and antibiotics, gain entry to the inner globe through the highly permeable sclera (Fig. 367).

Episcleritis is a localized, elevated, and tender, but not usually painful, inflammation of the episclera (Fig. 314). It lasts for weeks and may be suppressed with a mild topical steroid if itchy or uncomfortable. It is often a non-specific immune response but, infrequently, occurs in gout, syphilis, rheumatoid arthritis, and gastrointestinal disorders.

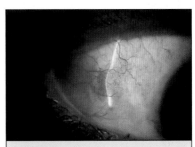

Fig 314 Episcleritis has a 60% occurrence rate.

Scleritis is a relatively uncommon severe inflammation of the sclera that may cause blindness. Unlike episcleritis, it is often painful, and the deep, engorged vessels do not blanch when topical phenylephrine 10% is instilled. A quarter of the cases are associated with systemic immune or infectious diseases such as systemic lupus erythematosus, rheumatoid arthritis, Lyme disease, tuberculosis, and syphilis, to name a few. Anterior scleritis is associated with visible engorgement of vessels deep to the conjunctiva (Fig. 315).

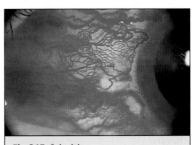

Fig 315 Scleritis.

Posterior scleritis causes choroidal effusions (Fig. 351) and even retinal detachments. Systemic corticosteroids, antimetabolites, or anti-infective drugs are usually required. Blood tests may include angiotensin-converting enzyme (ACE) for sarcoidosis; antinuclear antibody (ANA) for lupus; c-antineutrophil cytoplasmic antibody (c-ANCA) for Wegener's granulomatosis; p-antineutrophil cytoplasmic antibody (p-ANCA) for arteritis; fluorescent treponemal antibody (FTA)-ABS and Venereal Disease Research Laboratory (VDRL) test for syphilis; ELISA Western blot for Lyme disease; rheumatoid factor (RF) for rheumatoid arthritis; and C-reactive protein and erythrocyte sedimentation rate for non-specific systemic inflammation. Oral NSAIDS and steroids are the mainstays of treatment (Table 14, p. 145)

A blue sclera is due to increased scleral transparency, which allows choroidal pigment to be seen. It occurs normally in newborns, and abnormally in osteogenesis imperfecta (blue sclera with brittle bones), or following scleritis in rheumatoid arthritis (Fig. 316).

A staphyloma is a localized prolapse of bluish uveal tissue into thinned sclera. It occurs in rheumatoid arthritis, pathologic myopia (often over 10 D), or trauma (Fig. 317).

Jaundice, or icterus, refers to yellowing of the skin or sclera due to increased levels of bilirubin (Fig. 318). Because the elastin in the sclera has an increased affinity for bilirubin, it is often the first symptom of the condition. Total bilirubin is usually 0.3–1.0 mg/dL in adults and 1.0–12 mg/dL in newborns. Icterus first becomes toxic in adults above 12 mg/ dL. Above this level, newborns could develop mental retardation; a condition called kernicterus.

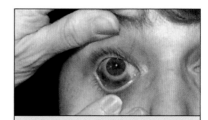

Fig 316 Rheumatoid arthritis causing thin sclera with visible underlying choroid.

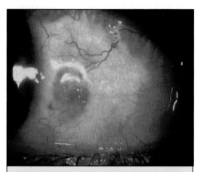

Fig 317 Staphyloma is a weakening of the sclera causing a bulging of the wall of the eye (ectasia). It is most often due to pathologic myopia, trauma, elevated eye pressure, or inflammatory damage from scleritis.

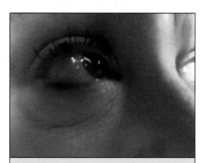

Fig 318 Jaundice (icterus): yellow skin and sclera due to elevated bilirubin.

Chapter 7
Glaucoma

The only way you know if you have glaucoma is to get tested.

Glaucoma is a disease of the optic nerve due to elevated intraocular pressure pressing on the blood supply to the nerve or on the ganglion cell axon disrupting axonal transport. Damage to the nerve causes loss of vision that is usually irreversible.

Intraocular pressure is maintained by a balance between aqueous inflow and outflow. The aqueous produced by the ciliary body processes (Figs 319 and 321) passes from the posterior chamber (the space behind the iris) through the pupil into the anterior chamber (Fig. 319). Most then drains through the trabecular meshwork through the venous canal of Schlemm and exits the eye through the episcleral veins. About 15% passes through the ciliary body and sclera (Figs 321 and 322) before exiting the eye through the scleral and episcleral venous plexus (uveoscleral pathway).

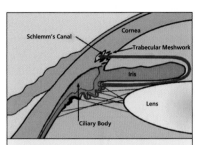

Fig 319 Aqueous flow from ciliary body to Schlemm's canal. *Source:* Courtesy of Pfizer Pharmaceuticals.

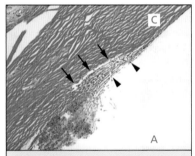

Fig 320 Histology showing Schlemm's canal (arrows), trabecular meshwork (arrowheads), aqueous (A), and cornea (C).

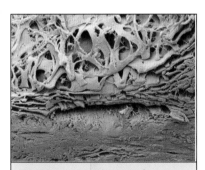

Fig 322 Microscopic view of trabecular meshwork that overlies Schlemm's canal. Obstructions at this meshwork prevent aqueous from reaching the canal, causing elevation of pressure.

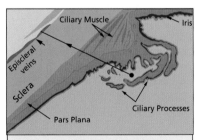

Fig 321 Uveoscleral outflow of aqueous produced by ciliary processes exits the eye by passing through ciliary body muscle and sclera to reach the episcleral veins.

Manual for Eye Examination and Diagnosis, Tenth Edition. Mark W. Leitman.
© 2021 John Wiley & Sons Ltd. Published 2021 by John Wiley & Sons Ltd.

Glaucoma vs. glaucoma suspect

Normal intraocular pressure is 10–20 mmHg and should be measured at different times of day as there is a circadian rhythm. Pressure 28 mmHg or more is usually treated regardless of other findings. Treat pressures of 20–27 mmHg when there is loss of vision, a family history of glaucoma, damage to the optic nerve as evidenced by disk pallor with increased cupping and thinning of the ganglion nerve fiber thickness (Figs 334–343). Patients with pressures of 20–27 mmHg without other suspicious findings of glaucoma are called *glaucoma suspects*. They are followed with more frequent visits than usual, with monitoring of eye pressure, visual fields, and optic nerve changes. When treatment is started, pressures are usually kept below 20 mmHg, which most often prevents loss in vision. However, some patients may lose vision even when pressures are kept in the high teens. These eyes require further lowering of pressure to the low teens and such patients have the condition referred to as low-pressure or normal-tension glaucoma. It is present up to 90% of Asians with glaucoma and in less than 50% of glaucoma patients worldwide.

Several instruments can be used to indirectly measure intraocular pressure by indenting the cornea, as follows.

1 A Goldmann applanation tonometer (Fig. 323) is the most accurate instrument for this purpose. It is used in conjunction with a slit lamp, and requires the use of anesthetic drops and fluorescein dye.

2 The Schiötz tonometer and Tono-Pen are portable instruments (Fig. 324) that also indent the anesthetized cornea and are used for bedside measurements.

3 The air-puff tonometer tests the pressure by blowing a puff of air at the eye. It is used by technicians since it does not require eye drops or corneal contact, but is more uncomfortable and slightly less accurate.

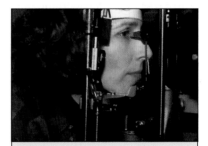

Fig 323 Goldmann tonometer: The gold standard for measuring eye pressure.

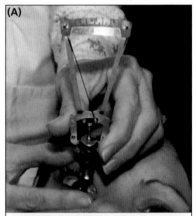

(A)

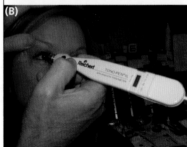

(B)

Fig 324 Portable tonometers: (A) Schiötz tonometer. (B) Tono-Pen applanation tonometer.

With all three instruments, the tonometric pressure reading is only an estimate of the real pressure. A thick cornea requires extra force to indent and, therefore, gives a falsely elevated reading, and the opposite is true with thin corneas. To better approximate the real pressure—especially in glaucoma suspects where exactitude is important—an ultrasonic pachymeter is used to measure the central corneal thickness. A conversion factor for corneal thickness then adjusts the tonometric reading upward with thin corneas or downward with thick corneas (Fig. 325). With scarred distorted corneas or uncooperative patients, finger-tip assessment may yield a gross evaluation.

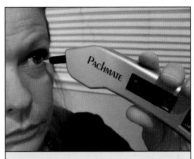

Fig 325 Measurement of corneal thickness with ultrasonic pachymeter.

The iridocorneal angle

Most aqueous leaves the eye by entering the trabecular meshwork (Fig. 326) which is the tan to dark brown band at the angle between the cornea and iris. It then exits the eye after entering the canal of Schlemm, which is a 360° circular tube leading into the scleral and episcleral venous plexus. The angle between the iris and the cornea is normally 15–45° and can be estimated with a slit lamp (Figs 328 and 329), but a goniolens (Figs 330 and 331) is more accurate. In open-angle glaucoma, the trabecular meshwork is obstructed, whereas in narrow-angle glaucoma, the space between

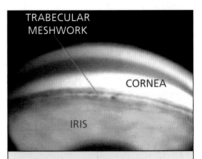

Fig 326 Normal trabecular meshwork: grade 4 angle as seen in a goniolens.

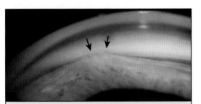

Fig 327 Peripheral anterior synechiae ↑ are adhesions between the iris and cornea partially obstructing the trabecular meshwork sometimes due to previous episodes of narrow angle glaucoma or iritis. It could reduce aqueous outflow. Distinguish from posterior synechiae which are adhesions between iris and lens (Figs 397–399). *Source*: Courtesy of Eyerounds.org, University of Iowa.

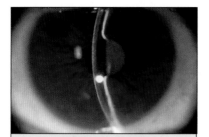

Fig 328 The anterior chamber is the space between the iris and cornea. It is shallow in a short hyperopic eye causing a narrow angle between the surfaces.

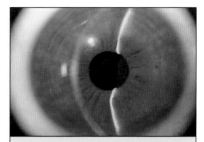

Fig 329 Deep anterior chamber with wide open angle in long myopic eye.

the iris and cornea is too narrow, so aqueous cannot reach the trabecular meshwork. A narrow angle at risk of closing is graded 0–2 (see Fig. 333). Angles of grade 3 or 4 are considered wide open with no chance of closing.

The optic disk (optic papilla)

The disk is the circular junction where the ganglion cell axons exit the eye, pick up a myelin sheath, and become the optic nerve (Figs 334–337, 339, and 474). The lamina cribrosa is the perforated continuation of the scleral wall of the eye that allows passage of

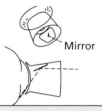

Mirror

Fig 330 Trabecular meshwork seen with a goniolens at the slit lamp (see Fig. 332).

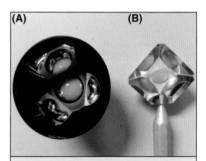

(A)   (B)

Fig 331 (A) Goldmann and (B) Zeiss gonioscope lenses used to examine the angle of the eye at the slit lamp. The Goldmann lens also gives precise magnified visualization of the optic disk.

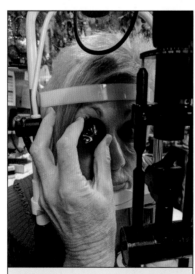

Fig 332 Examination of angle with Goldmann lens at slit lamp.

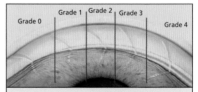

Grade 0   Grade 1   Grade 2   Grade 3   Grade 4

Fig 333 Grading angle by progressive widening from 0 to 4. *Source:* Courtesy of Pfizer Pharmaceuticals.

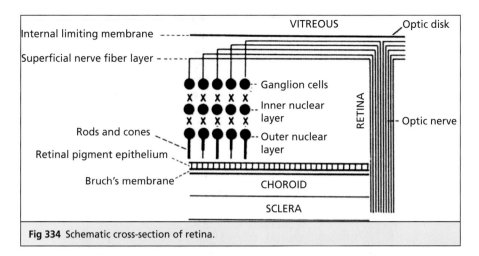

Fig 334 Schematic cross-section of retina.

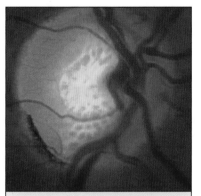

Fig 335 Lamina cribrosa forms the floor of optic disk. Note perforations for passage of nerves and blood vessels. *Source*: Courtesy of University of Iowa, Eyerounds.org.

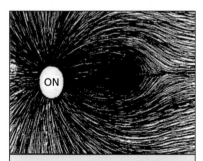

Fig 336 Drawing of retinal nerve fiber layer with 1.2 million ganglion cell axons converging to make up the optic nerve (ON).

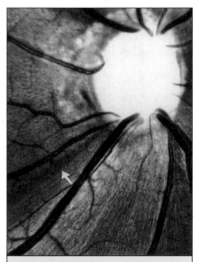

Fig 337 "Red-free" photograph of glaucomatous cupping and loss of retinal nerve fiber layer (white arrow). The dark area with loss of striations is pathognomonic of fiber loss if it fans out and widens further from disk. *Source*: Courtesy of Michael P. Kelly.

the retina ganglion cell axons and the central retinal artery and veins to exit the globe (Fig. 335). A central depression within it forms the optic cup that is usually less than one-third the disk diameter, although larger cups can be normal (Fig. 340).

Signs of nerve fiber damage

As pressure damages the nerve:

1 cup/disk ratio increases (Fig. 340),
2 cup becomes more excavated and often unequal in the two eyes,
3 vessels shift nasally (Fig. 340D),
4 disk margin loses capillaries and turns pale; flame hemorrhages on the disk (Fig. 340C) are associated with more rapid loss of central visual field, as opposed to the usual peripheral loss in glaucoma,
5 diffuse loss of retinal nerve fiber layer (Figs 337 and 343).

The optic disk changes can be followed by accurate drawings, photographs, or OCT or GDx testing (Figs 338, 339, 341, and 343). Retinal nerve fiber layer thickness is usually measured around the optic disk (less often the macula) with OCT or GDx. It is most useful in detecting early stages of glaucoma before visual field loss becomes evident. A 5 μm progressive loss of thickness between tests is significant. (A red blood cell has a diameter of 7 μm.)

Visual field defects pathognomonic of glaucoma (Fig. 344)

1 Bjerrum's scotoma extends nasally from the blind spot in an arc.
2 Island defects could enlarge into a Bjerrum's scotoma.
3 Constricted fields occur before loss of central vision.
4 Ronne's nasal step is loss of peripheral nasal field above or below the horizontal.

The diagnosis and treatment of open-angle glaucoma should initially be made before visual field loss based on eye pressure, optic nerve findings, nerve fiber layer thickness,

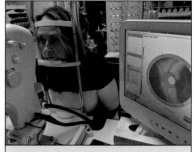

Fig 338 Optical coherent tomography (OCT) performed in office showing normally thicker nerve fiber layer inferiorly and superiorly.

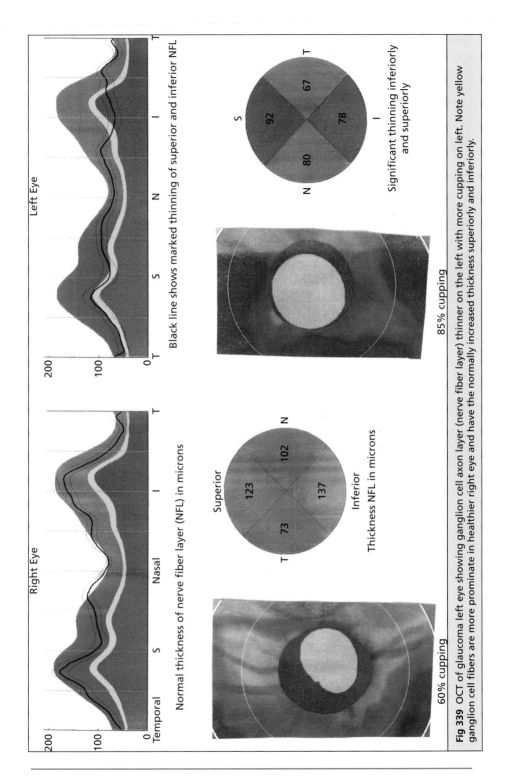

Fig 339 OCT of glaucoma left eye showing ganglion cell axon layer (nerve fiber layer) thinner on the left with more cupping on left. Note yellow ganglion cell fibers are more prominate in healthier right eye and have the normally increased thickness superiorly and inferiorly.

Right Eye

Left Eye

200

100

0

Temporal S Nasal S I T

Normal thickness of nerve fiber layer (NFL) in microns

200

100

0

T S N S I T

Black line shows marked thinning of superior and inferior NFL

Superior

Thickness NFL in microns

Inferior

N

102

123 137

73

T

60% cupping

Significant thinning inferiorly and superiorly

T

67

S 92 78 I

80

N

85% cupping

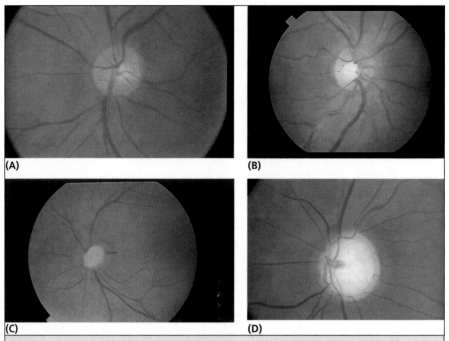

Fig 340 Optic cup/disk ratio (A) C/D = 0.25; (B) C/D = 0.40; (C) C/D = 0.70 with hemorrhage; (D) C/D = 0.90. Some people have normally enlarged optic sups from birth. These eyes should be monitored as they age since they could be more susceptible to ischemic damage from lower pressures.

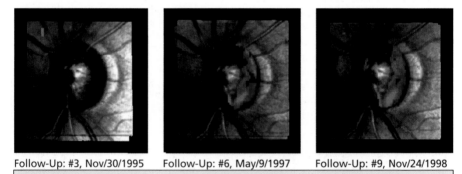

Follow-Up: #3, Nov/30/1995   Follow-Up: #6, May/9/1997   Follow-Up: #9, Nov/24/1998

Fig 341 Scanning laser optic disk tomography (OCT) with red color indicating progressive cupping over a 3-year period. *Source*: Courtesy of Heidelberg Engineering, Inc.

and family history. If one waits for visual field loss, 20% of the nerve fiber layer may have already been lost.

The goal is to reduce pressure below 20 mmHg, or at least to a level where there is no further loss of visual field, increase in cupping

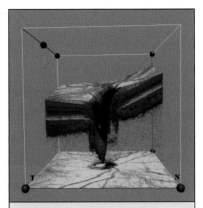

Fig 342 Three-dimensional OCT using high-speed ultra-high resolution to create multiple cross-sectional images of optic nerve cupping. *Source*: Courtesy of Elizabeth Affel, OCT-C, Wills Eye Hospital.

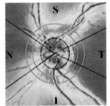

Healthy retinal nerve fiber layer

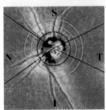

Moderate retinal nerve fiber loss

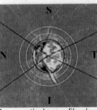

Severe retinal nerve fiber loss

Thickness Map Legend (microns)

0   20   40   60   80   100 120 140 160 180 200

Fig 343 Color-coded GDx scanning laser polarimetry showing loss of thicker (yellow) nerve fiber layer over several years. It should be noted that the nerve fiber layer is normally thickest inferiorly then superiorly, followed by nasally, and then temporally. This can be remembered by the acronym *ISN'T*. *Source*: Courtesy of Carl Zeiss Meditec., Inc.

or loss of nerve fiber. Each patient should have a target pressure which is set at a lower pressure in severe glaucoma, or, if optic nerve damage continues to progress. Maintenance of pressures in the high teens is usually sufficient. Continued progression of visual field loss and nerve fiber damage occurring with pressures controlled in the high teens requires further pressure lowering, often to the low teens. This is referred to as *low-tension glaucoma*. Pressure-lowering treatment requires a combination of one or more medications; one from each of the classes (Table 11, p. 126) or require the addition of a surgical procedure.

Medical treatment (Table 11)

Initial treatment of open angle glaucoma usually starts with eye drops. Be sure the drops are being used properly. Only 20% of the eye drop is retained on the surface of the eye with most of it running onto the cheek or into the nose. Only half of the 20% remains in the eye after 4 minutes and only 3.4% remains after 10 minutes. Therefore, one should wait at least 10 minutes before administering a second drop. The effectiveness of a drop is

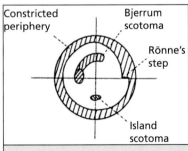

Fig 344 Visual field defects in glaucoma.

Table 11 Common glaucoma medications and side effects.

Action	Class	Chemical name	Trade name	Concentration	Dosage	Comment
↓Aqueous secretion by ciliary body processes	Beta-blocker	Timolol (G)	Timoptic Betimol	0.25 and 0.5% eye drops	BID	Slows heart rate Aggravates respiratory conditions Betoptic is cardioselective with the fewest systemic side effects
		Timoptic gel	Timoptic XE	0.25 and 0.5% eye drops	QD	
		Betaxolol (G)	Betoptic S	0.25% eye drops	BID	
			Timoptic	1/2 PF eye drops	Single dose ampules	
	Carbonic anhydrase inhibitor	Dorzolamide (G)	Trusopt	2% eye drops	TID	Could suppress bone marrow
	Topical	Brinzolamide	Azopt	1% eye drops	TID	
	Oral	Acetazolamide (G)	Diamox	250 mg tablet 500 mg tablet	QID BID	Could suppress bone marrow
↑Uveoscleral outflow (Fig. 321)	Prostaglandin analogue	Latanoprost (G) (most commonly used and least expensive, 56 cents per drop)	Xalatan	0.005% eye drops	HS	Darkening and lengthening of eyelashes with hyperpigmentation of iris and periocular (eyelid) skin, loss of orbital fat (Figs 11–13)
		Travoprost (G)	Travatan Z	0.004% eye drops	HS	
		Bimatoprost	Lumigan	0.01% eye drops	HS	
		Tafloprost(PF)	Zioptan	0.0015% eye drops	HS	Preservative free ampules (No bottle)

Action	Class	Chemical name	Trade name	Concentration	Dosage	Comment
↑Outflow trabecular meshwork (Fig. 319)	Cholinergic	Pilocarpine (G)	Pilocar	0.5–0.6% eye drops	QID	Retinal detachment cataracts, small pupil, brow ache
	Rho kinase inhibitor	Rhopressa	Netarsudil	0.02% eye drops	QD	Conjunctival injection, corneal lipid deposits
↓Aqueous secretion and ↑ uveoscleral outflow	Alpha-adrenergic agonist	Brimonidine (G)	Alphagan P	0.01, 0.15 & 0.2%	TID	Frequent allergy
↑Uveoscleral and trabecular meshwork outflow	Prostaglandin analogue with nitrous oxide release	Latanoprostene	Vyzulta	0.024% eye drops	HS	Nitric oxide ingredient reduces IOP an additional 2 mm over other prostaglandins but is expensive
Combination Glaucoma Medications (convenient)						
		Netarsudil and Latanoprost	Rocklatan	0.02 and 0.005% eye drops	HS	Expensive
		Brimonidine and Brinzolamide	Simbrinza	0.2 and 1% eye drops	TID	
		Timolol and Dorzolomide (G,PF)	Cosopt	0.5 and 2% eye drops	BID	Least expensive
		Brimonidine and Timolol	Combigan	0.2 and 0.5% eye drops	BID	

Generic (G) or preservative-free (PF) available.

increased by closing the eyelids which stops the pumping action of the blink and by applying digital pressure to the punctal area (Fig. 151). The American Glaucoma Society does not yet recommend marijuana to treat glaucoma.

Surgical procedures for open-angle glaucoma

Unfortunately, up to 60% of patients are non-compliant in using their drops on schedule, especially when using more than one drop. Always ask whether drops were used before their present visit. If properly used medications do not control the pressure, surgery can be performed. Procedures are first directed at increasing aqueous outflow, or less often, at reducing aqueous secretion. Selective laser trabeculoplasty (SLT) using a Nd:YAG laser or argon laser (ALT) applied to the trabecular meshwork increase outflow (Figs 345 and 346) and are usually the first surgical procedures to be tried. Some doctors are recommending SLT before treatment with eye drops, especially when cost or inconvenience of instilling drops are a problem. SLT can be repeated on the same area of trabecular meshwork more than once if needed, unlike the argon technique, and usually lowers pressure by 20% with the effect lasting 1–5 years. The latest 2020 study shows the pressure lowering effect may only last an average of 3 years.

If pressure is still too high, a surgical hole is created at the limbus (trabeculectomy) to drain aqueous through the sclera and under the conjunctiva (Figs 347–349). This has been the gold standard go to procedure for large elevations of pressure. After gently separating the conjunctiva and tenons fascia from the underlying sclera, a triangle of half-thickness sclera is dissected toward the limbus. A small window of the remaining sclera is excised to create an opening into the anterior chamber. The flap of sclera is partially closed followed by secure closure of overlying conjunctiva and tenons. The trabeculectomy could be repeated if the fistula closes, most often due to scarring of the episcleral flap. To

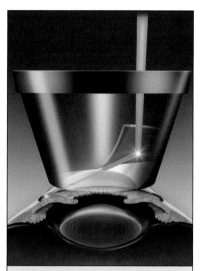

Fig 345 SLT trabeculoplasty requires a reflecting mirror on the eye to visualize and focus the laser on the trabecular meshwork hidden from direct view.

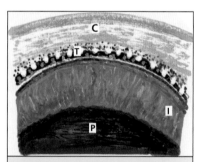

Fig 346 Drawing of SLT trabeculoplasty. Up to 100 shots (causing bubble formation) may be applied to pigmented trabecular meshwork around the entire 360° circumference. There were so far no sight-threatening complications. It increases aqueous outflow through the trabecular meshwork. C, cornea; T, trabecular meshwork; I, iris; P, pupil.

help prevent scarring and closure of the fistula, an anti-fibrotic such as Mitomycin C 0.02% may be topically applied to the area at the time of surgery. If still unsuccessful, a tube could be implanted connecting the anterior chamber with the subconjunctival space (Fig. 353). One complication of these two procedures is that it exposes the interior of the eye to infection since only the overlying conjunctiva protects the inner globe (Fig. 352). Another complication is hypotony due to

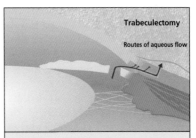

Fig 347 Surgical trabeculectomy showing aqueous flow from ciliary body through iridectomy and scleral tunnel. It exits eye under conjunctiva. *Source*: Courtesy of Pfizer Pharmaceuticals.

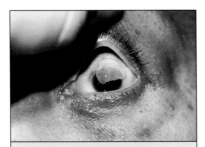

Fig 349 A trabeculectomy is a surgically created fistula from anterior chamber to subconjunctival space. This bleb was too large and irritated the cornea and needs to be revised. *Source*: Courtesy of Steven Brown, MD, and *Arch. Ophthalmol.*, Nov. 1999, Vol. 1, p. 156. Copyright 1999, American Medical Association. All rights reserved.

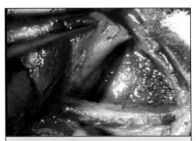

Fig 348 Dissection of sclera towards the limbus. A window of the sclera is then removed for entry into Schlemm's canal.

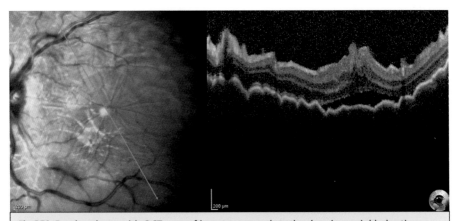

Fig 350 Fundus photo with OCT scan of hypotony maculopathy showing wrinkled retina. Folds (stria) may also occur in the cornea (Fig. 267). A target pressure of 6 mmHg or more is usually sought. Compare OCT with normal (Fig. 463). *Source*: Courtesy of University of Iowa, Eyerounds.org.

overfiltration or wound leak. The hypotony could cause corneal folds (stroma) (Fig. 267) edema of the macula (Figs 350 and 351) and effusion of fluid into the choroid (choroidal). Leaks through the conjunctiva are identified with the Seidel test in which fluorescein dye is placed on the suspected site. Cobalt blue light is used to show the green-stained stream of leaking aqueous. Excessive egress of fluid occurs in about 15% of trabeculectomies and 5% of cases using drainage devices (stents) (Fig. 353). In a 2020 study comparing 117 trabeculectomy surgeries with 125 tube shunts, there was no significant difference in the pressure-lowering effect after 3 years.

Complications of trabeculectomy led to development of minimally invasive glaucoma surgeries (MIGS). In one technique, two tiny titanium stents (iStent) that are passed through a single corneal wound penetrating the obstructed trabecular meshwork with side ports opening into Schlemm's canal (Fig. 354). They are placed 2–3 clock hours apart. It is often done as a secondary procedure during cataract surgery since the eye is already entered. It is the smallest device ever approved by the FDA.

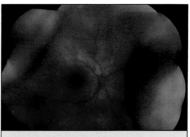

Fig 351 Very low pressure (hypotony) or posterior scleritis can cause a choroidal effusion with a serous collection of fluid referred to as a *choroidal*. It causes an elevation of the retina which can be confused with a retinal detachment. Its smooth, bulbous, and sometimes 360° presence together with hypotony helps differentiate it from a retinal detachment (RD) (Fig. 578). The RD is often wrinkled with a retinal hole and normal eye pressure.

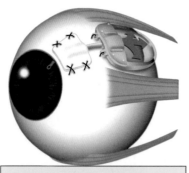

Fig 353 Ahmed glaucoma valve. Tube in anterior chamber drains aqueous to subconjunctival space. To prevent erosion through the conjunctiva, the implant could be covered with a graft made up of commercially available human cornea, sclera, or pericardium. A tube too close to the corneal endothelium has been shown to be a risk for development of corneal edema. *Source*: Courtesy of New World Medical, Inc.

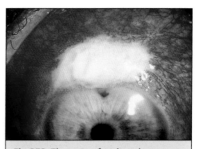

Fig 352 The rate of trabeculectomy bleb-related infection is about 1.5% after 2 years, but is reported up to 8% when followed for longer periods. This conjunctival bleb was too thin and got infected. The interior of this eye is at risk of endophthalmitis, which could cause blindness. *Source*: Courtesy of Donald L. Bendenz and *Arch. Ophthalmol.*, Aug. 1999, Vol. 117, p. 1010. Copyright 1999, American Medical Association. All rights reserved.

Another MIGS technique uses a surgical instrument called a *trabectome*. It uses electrical pulses to vaporize about 90° of diseased trabecular tissue that obstructs access to Schlemm's canal (Figs 355–357). The trabecular meshwork may also be excised with the Kahook Dual Blade (Figs 358 and 359). The removal of trabecular meshwork creates a cleft more resistant to closure than simple incision (goniotomy) which was previously a mainstay treatment for congenital glaucoma.

The surgeries discussed here increase aqueous outflow from the eye. Another strategy is

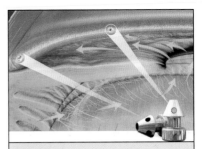

Fig 354 The titanium iStent Trabecular Micro-Bypass Stent (Glaukos) drains aqueous into Schlemm's canal from the anterior chamber effectively bypassing the blocked trabecular meshwork.

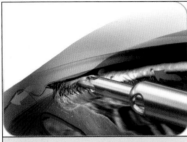

Fig 355 Trabectome unroofing Schlemm's canal. *Source:* Invented by Roy Chuck, MD, and George Baerveldt, MD, Albert Einstein Medical School.

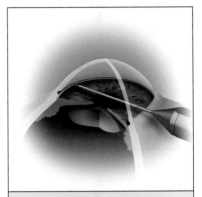

Fig 358 Kahook Dual Blade enters cornea avoiding conjunctiva. *Source:* Courtesy of New World Medical.

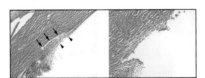

Fig 356 Trabectome removal of trabecular meshwork (↑↑) to expose Schlemm's canal ↑↑↑.

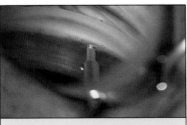

Fig 357 Photo of trabectome.

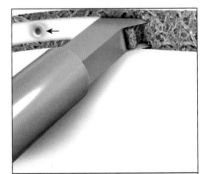

Fig 359 Kahook Dual Blade used to remove 3–4 hours of trabecular meshwork—also note previously inserted stent ⊠. *Source:* Courtesy of New World Medical.

to surgically reduce aqueous inflow by destroying some of the ciliary processes. To accomplish this, transscleral "cryo" or laser therapy may be applied to the area directly overlying the ciliary processes (Fig. 360)—endoscopic cyclophotocoagulation may be performed by entering the eye, often during cataract surgery, and destroying the ciliary processes with a laser utilizing direct visualization (Fig. 361).

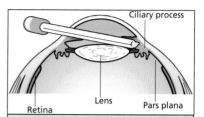

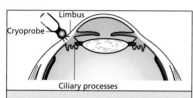

Fig 360 Transscleral cryotherapy is applied for less than 20 seconds to 180° of sclera 1 mm posterior to the limbus. Transscleral diode laser may also be used to destroy part of the ciliary body.

Fig 361 Endoscopic cyclophotocoagulation for partial destruction of aqueous-secreting ciliary processes. One probe consisting of a light source, laser, and camera is usually inserted into the eye near the corneal limbus, although a pars plana site may be used. Anywhere from 170° to 280° is usually treated. Most common side effects may include iritis and temporary decrease in vision.

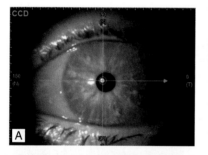

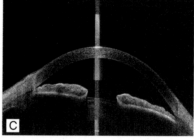

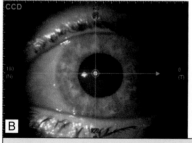

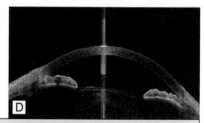

Fig 362 OCT of closed angle after pupil dilation (see Table 6, p. 53). Source: Courtesy of Dr. Jorge Vila-Artega and Dr. Isabel Pascual Camps, Clinica Vila, Valencia, Spain.

vw. **A** Small pupil   **Fig. C** Open Angle
Fig. B Dilated pupil   **Fig. D** Closed angle afterdilation

Angle-closure glaucoma

Angle-closure glaucoma is less common than the previously discussed open-angle glaucoma, and its treatment is different (Table 12, p. 134). It usually occurs in hyperopic eyes that are short with crowded anterior segments. The iris in these eyes is closer to the cornea (Figs 328, 329, 362, and 364) commonly in hyperopic eyes with short axial length. The resulting narrow angle becomes even more narrow when the pupil becomes mid-dilated. In this position, there is maximum contact between the iris and lens, preventing the aqueous from reaching the anterior chamber and trabecular meshwork. This "pupillary block" traps aqueous behind the iris and pushes the iris forward even more until the angle is totally closed. The total closure of the angle causes a sudden elevation in pressure, often exceeding 60 mmHg. This pressure damages the pupil, causing it to remain fixed and dilated.

Symptoms include pain, blurred vision, halos, and nausea. Signs include a mid-dilated non-reactive pupil, and corneal edema, with venous engorgement of conjunctival vessels (Figs 363, 364, and 396).

Pupil dilation precipitating this attack may be caused by stimulation of the pupillary dilator muscle by adrenergic drugs, such as decongestants used to treat allergy, and phenylephrine, which dilates the pupil for the retinal exam. Stress or darkness may also cause a similar effect. Anticholinergic drops (Table 15, p. 147), used for pupil dilation and to treat iritis, block the pupillary sphincter muscle. Topamax (topiramate), used to treat epilepsy and prevent migraines, may also trigger this attack by causing ciliochoroidal effusions. This swelling pushes the iris anteriorly. Immediately discontinue the drug.

Treatment of angle-closure glaucoma first requires lowering of the pressure to break the attack and clear the cornea. It usually includes pilocarpine 1% to constrict the pupil and up to three other pressure-lowering types of eye drops. If the pressure still remains too high, a short-acting hyperosmotic agent such as

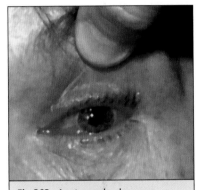

Fig 363 Acute angle-closure glaucoma with dilated pupil.

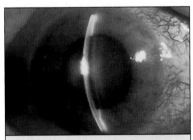

Fig 364 Angle closure glaucoma: As the eye pressure steadily rises above 35 mmHg it may cause pain which is not usually a symptom of glaucoma. This pressure may damage the pupillary sphincter muscle, and the corneal endothelium resulting in a fixed dilated pupil with corneal edema (see Table 12, p. 134).

Table 12 Common types of glaucoma.		
	Primary open-angle glaucoma	*Angle-closure glaucoma*
Occurrence	70% of all glaucomas	10% of all glaucomas
Etiology	Unknown obstruction in trabecular meshwork, usually inherited; increases with age	Closed-angle glaucoma increases with age and hyperopia
Symptoms	Usually asymptomatic	Red, painful eye; halos around lights; nausea
Signs	Elevated pressure Increased disk cupping Visual field defect OCT showing thinned nerve fiber layer (Fig. 339)	Markedly elevated pressure Steamy cornea Fixed, mid-dilated pupil Conjunctival injection

intravenous mannitol 20% or oral glycerin 50% may be administered. Both draw fluid out of the eye by increasing the osmolarity of the blood. Once the attack is arrested, the corneal edema may be further cleared with topical hypertonic 2% saline solution. Then, a laser iridotomy can be performed (Fig. 365). This allows aqueous to flow into the anterior chamber and bypass the pupillary block. It is often a permanent cure and the pupil may then be safely dilated. Lens extraction is an alternative when the iridotomy isn't successful. Prophylactic iridotomies to prevent an attack is indicated in patients with narrow angles, especially if they have peripheral anterior synechiae (PAS) present from previous attack (Fig. 327); a family history of angle closure; or if there is high eye pressure.

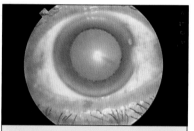

Fig 365 Nd: YAG laser peripheral iridotomy at 2 o'clock.

Less common types of glaucoma, called *secondary open-angle glaucoma*, could be caused by blockage of the trabecular meshwork by pigment (as in melanosis oculi) (Fig. 366), pseudoexfoliation (Fig. 368), hyphema (Fig. 369), or venous congestion due to orbital disease and cavernous sinus thrombosis or fistula. Patients with neovascularization of the iris (Figs 388 and 389) must not only be treated for elevation of pressure but also for the retinal ischemia causing it. Corticosteroids could elevate eye pressure especially when used in high concenrations over prolonged periods of time. They are

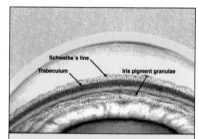

Fig 366 Pigment of dispersion syndrome causing secondary glaucoma.

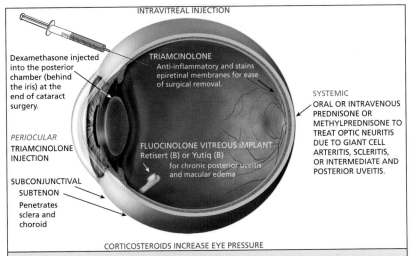

INTRAVITREAL INJECTION

Dexamethasone injected into the posterior chamber (behind the iris) at the end of cataract surgery.

TRIAMCINOLONE
Anti-inflammatory and stains epiretinal membranes for ease of surgical removal.

PERIOCULAR
TRIAMCINOLONE INJECTION

SUBCONJUNCTIVAL
SUBTENON
Penetrates sclera and choroid

FLUOCINOLONE VITREOUS IMPLANT
Retisert (B) or Yutiq (B)
for chronic posterior uveitis and macular edema

SYSTEMIC
ORAL OR INTRAVENOUS PREDNISONE OR METHYLPREDNISONE TO TREAT OPTIC NEURITIS DUE TO GIANT CELL ARTERITIS, SCLERITIS, OR INTERMEDIATE AND POSTERIOR UVEITIS.

CORTICOSTEROIDS INCREASE EYE PRESSURE

Fig 367 There are a number of types of steroids. Corticosteroids are one type. Cortisol derives it's name from it's site of production in the cortex of the adrenal gland on top of kidney. Synthetic equivalents shown above have similar molecular structures, i.e. 3 hexane rings and 1 pentane ring. They however differ in their anti-inflammatory potencies and duration of action. Prescribers of corticosteroids without the ability to measure eye pressure should contact an eye doctor to determine how often it should be measured. All could raise intraocular pressure, some more than others (Brand B, Generic G).

used extensively in all forms in treating eye disease (Fig. 367). Other common uses include oral preparations for treatment of asthma, COPD, allergy, autoimmune disease, sarcoidosis and cancers such as lymphoma and multiple myeloma to name just a few. Your history taking should include the frequently used over-the counter nasal sprays used for allergic rhinitis, and sinusitis which together with creams to treat dermatitis often go unmentioned.

Trauma could cause glaucoma by tearing the iris at its insertion on the ciliary body. Gonioscopy may reveal angle recession (Figs 369 and 370), in which the iris insertion is torn posteriorly, exposing a wide band of darkly pigmented ciliary body. Often, there is associated bleeding in the anterior chamber referred to as a *hyphema*. Complications of hyphema include rebleeds, associated retinal damage, and glaucoma. Rx: bilateral patch and absolute bedrest for 5 days. Patients should be monitored indefinitely because about 10% ultimately develop glaucoma.

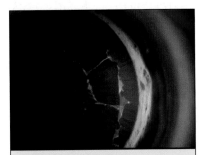

Fig 368 Pseudoexfoliation is identified by white flakes on the anterior lens capsule, pupillary margin, zonules, and trabecular meshwork. It is relatively common and is associated with a 25% incidence of glaucoma. The weakened zonules could complicate cataract surgery since there is less support for the lens implant (Figs 453 and 454). *Source*: Courtesy of Rhonda Curtis, CRA, COT, Washington University Medical School, St. Louis, MO, and *J. Ophthalmic Photogr*.

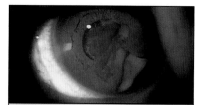

Fig 369 Hyphema with large iris disinsertion (dialysis) from its root causing angle damage and obstruction of by red blood cells.

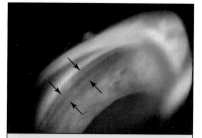

Fig 370 Angle recessed posteriorly following traumatic hyphema. The recessed angle is seen as a wide, dark band between the cornea and the iris (↑). These patients may initially have normal eye pressure, but should be monitored for future onset of glaucoma.

Congenital glaucoma is fortunately rare, but must be suspected since routine office eye pressure measurements are difficult, if not impossible, in infants and young children. Clues to arouse suspicion are squinting, tearing, an enlarged globe (buphthalmos) (Fig. 372), and corneal edema. The latter may cause a subtle loss of a normally shiny, clear corneal surface (Fig. 371), which is due to the damaging effect of the pressure on the corneal endothelium. The most common surgical procedure for congenital glaucoma is a goniotomy in which an incision is made through the obstructed trabecular meshwork.

One type of juvenile glaucoma occurs in Sturge–Weber syndrome (Fig. 199), in which there is angiomatosis of the face and meninges with cerebral calcifications and seizures. Extreme caution must be exercised during any ocular surgery on these patients to avoid bleeding in their highly vascularized eye. The treatment of pediatric glaucoma is primarily surgical because medications are often ineffective and poorly tolerated in the long run.

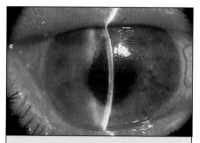

Fig 371 Very high pressure, often over 35 mmHg damage the pumping action of the corneal endothelium causing a cloudy, edematous cornea.

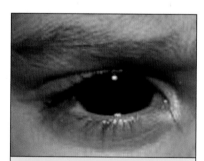

Fig 372 Congenital glaucoma in an 8-month-old, with squinting, an enlarged globe, and subtle corneal edema causing an obscured view of the iris. *Source*: Courtesy of Karen Joos, MD, PhD, Vanderbilt Eye Institute.

Chapter 8
Uvea

Functionally, melanin serves as a protection against UV radiation.

The uvea (Fig. 373) is composed of the iris, ciliary body, and choroid. All three are contiguous and pigmented with melanocytes.

The iris is a diaphragm that changes the size of the pupil by the action of the sympathetic dilator muscle and the cholinergic constrictor muscle (Fig. 125).

Brushfield spots are normally occurring small, white-to-brown elevations on the peripheral iris, more common in hazel or blue iris and in Down's syndrome (Fig. 375).

The ciliary body (Figs 374, 376, and 378) is made up of four clinically significant parts, as follows:

1 The anterior region serves as the site for insertion of the iris, and includes the trabecular meshwork (Figs 319–322).
2 The ciliary processes secrete the aqueous (Figs 319, 373, and 376) that nourishes the lens and cornea while maintaining intraocular pressure.
3 The smooth muscle changes the focus of the lens by contracting and decreasing tension on the zonules (Figs 376 and 377), and provides the site—the uveoscleral pathway—for aqueous to exit the eye.
4 The flat avascular pars plana serves as the best location to surgically enter the eye for intravitreal injections and vitreoretinal surgery (Figs 373, 460, 526, 527, and 553–555).

The choroid has the highest tissue blood flow and least oxygen extraction of any tissue in the body supplying 70% of the blood flow to the eye. Its purpose is to nourish the retina, which has one of the highest metabolic rates of any tissue in the body. Unlike the tree-like

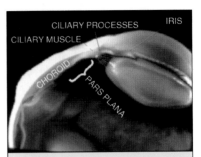

Fig 373 Uvea. *Source:* Courtesy of Stephen McCormick.

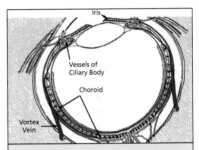

Fig 374 The uvea is made up of the iris, ciliary body, and choroid. *Source:* Courtesy of Pfizer Pharmaceuticals.

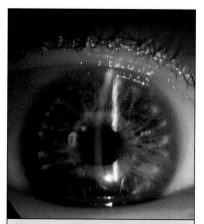

Fig 375 Brushfield spots are lightly colored spots on the iris common to Down's syndrome and light irides. *Source*: Courtesy of University of Iowa, Eyerounds.org.

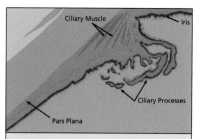

Fig 376 Ciliary body. *Source*: Courtesy of Pfizer Pharmaceuticals.

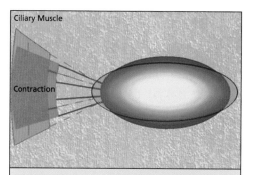

Fig 377 Ciliary muscle contraction lessens tension on zonules causing the lens to become more convex which changes its focus from distance to near. *Source*: Courtesy of Pfizer Pharmaceuticals.

branching of the retinal vessels, the choroidal circulation appears to crisscross in a tigroid-like appearance (Fig. 378). It is most easily visualized in advanced dry age-related macular degeneration (also called geographic AMD) after the retinal pigment layer disappears (Fig. 518) or in albinism where the retinal pigment is never fully developed (Fig. 540). The choriocapillaris may develop abnormal neovascularization in wet age-related macular degeneration, pathologic myopia,

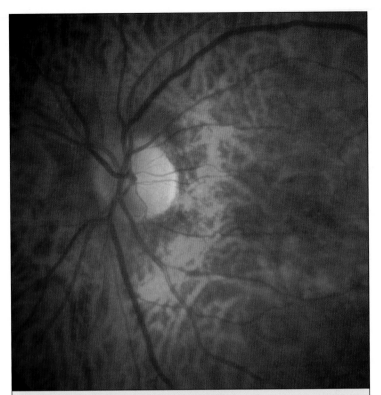

Fig 378 Tigroid fundus with clearly visible, lightly pigmented choroidal vasculature. *Source*: Courtesy of Elliot Davidoff, MD.

and presumed histoplasmosis (Figs 519–521 and 524).

Malignant uveal tumors

Six percent of metastatic tumors from elsewhere in the body go to the eye and the choroid is the most common ocular site. The primary site is most commonly the breast or lung. A melanocyte tumor is the most common primary intraocular malignancy. It is unilateral and develops from the choroid (Figs 379–384) in 85% of cases, the ciliary body in 9%, and the iris in 6% (Figs 313, 385, and 387). Ocular melanoma of the conjunctiva is the least common type (Figs 311 and 312). The risk may increase in fair-skinned

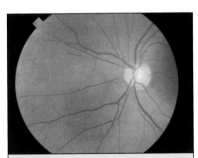

Fig 379 A flat benign choroidal nevus is present in 8% of Americans. Malignant transformation occurs in 1 in 9000/year.

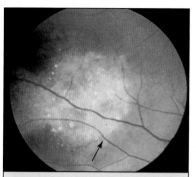

Fig 380 Elevated malignant choroidal melanoma. Note change in direction as artery rises over tumor (↑).

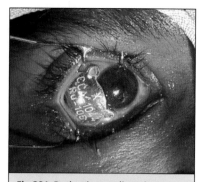

Fig 381 Ruthenium radioactive plaque sewn or glued to the episclera of the eye is usually left in place for about 4 days and is used to treat smaller intraocular tumors. It is referred to as brachytherapy. *Source*: Courtesy of Dr Santosh G. Honor and Dr Surbhi Joshi, Prasad Eye Institute, Hyderabad, India.

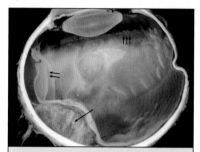

Fig 382 Gross section of malignant ↑ melanoma treated with removal of the eye (enucleation). Note retinal detachment ↑↑ and normally scalloped (serrated) junction of retina and pars plana ↑↑↑. The junction is, therefore, called the *ora serrata*. *Source*: Courtesy of University of Iowa, Eyerounds.com.

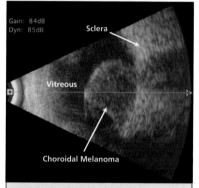

Fig 383 B-scan ultrasound of a malignant choroidal melanoma showing typical dome-shaped growth which helps to confirm the diagnosis. The scan also shows its size and whether it extends beyond the sclera which will determine the type of treatment. This eye, with its massive tumor, was enucleated.

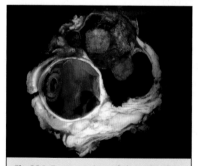

Fig 384 Exenteration of the orbit for malignant melanoma extending beyond the sclera. *Source*: J.J. Ross et al., *Br. J. Ophthalmol.*, 2010, Vol. 94, No. 5. Reproduced with permission of BMJ Publishing Group, Ltd.

people, ages 50–70, and with excess exposure to sunlight and with melanosis of conjunctiva and skin (Fig. 313). Unlike a benign nevus (Fig. 379), which is usually a more uniform gray color and flat (Fig. 379), choroidal tumors are elevated and usually slate gray, but may be white to black with yellow-gold and uneven pigmentation (Figs 380–384). This must be distinguished from metastatic carcinoma to the eye, which is also most common in the choroid, but is usually lighter in color. Primary and metastatic tumors of the eye are usually treated locally with external proton beam radiation or with a radioactive plaque brachytherapy (Fig. 381), both of which may preserve some vision. For larger tumors, the eye is sometimes removed by enucleation (Fig. 423). If the tumor extends beyond the globe and is life threatening, an exenteration of the orbit is required. This rarely performed surgery is disfiguring and destructive. It could necessitate removal of the orbital contents, the eyelids, orbital walls, and periorbital structures (Fig. 384). About 40% of uveal melanomas may metastasize. Metastatic tumors to the choroid, from elsewhere in the body, may be treated using laser photodynamic therapy with Verteporfin. It provides tumor control in 78% of eyes giving 20/40 or better vision in 66% of eyes.

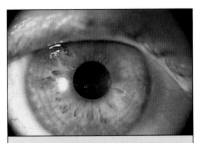

Fig 385 Benign iris freckle.

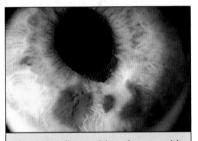

Fig 386 Malignant iris melanoma with elevated lesions and distorted pupil.

Patients with melanoma of the skin and elsewhere are often referred to eye physicians to rule out the eye as the primary site of origin of the tumor.

Benign iris freckles (Fig. 385) and nevi are common, whereas malignant iris melanoma (Figs 386 and 387) is rare. Lesions become more suspicious if they are growing, elevated, vascularized, distort the pupil, or cause inflammation, glaucoma, or cataracts.

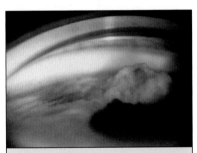

Fig 387 Gonioscopic view of elevated iris melanoma. *Source*: Courtesy of Michael P. Kelly.

Rubeosis iridis is a serious condition in which abnormal vessels grow on the surface of the iris (Figs 388 and 389) in response to ischemia associated with central retinal artery or vein occlusion, proliferative diabetic retinopathy, or carotid artery occlusive disease. Untreated, the neovascularization could cause end-stage

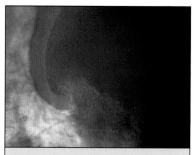

Fig 388 Rubeosis iridis with neovascularization.

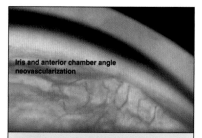

Fig 389 Rubeosis iridis. These abnormal iris blood vessels scar the angle of the eye. They most often result from ischemic retinal diseases such as proliferative diabetic retinopathy and central retinal artery or vein occlusion.

glaucoma, painful enough to require multiple glaucoma surgeries or rarely require removal of the eye (enucleation). Laser photocoagulation, or intravitreal anti-VEGF (vascular endothelial growth factor) injections often cause regression of iris vessels.

An iris coloboma (Fig. 390) is due to failure of embryonic tissue to fuse inferiorly. It may also involve the choroid, lens, and optic nerve.

Inflammation of the uvea (uveitis)

Inflammations of the uvea are categorized by location: A, anterior (iritis); B, intermediate involving the ciliary body (cyclitis); C. posterior (choroiditis); and D, panuveitis, involving all uveal structures. There are many possible causes (Table 16, p. 148) and sometimes no etiology is found. Treatments vary depending on the cause, the severity and the chronicity. Most often the go-to therapy includes corticosteroids but non-steroidals (NSAIDS), antimetabolites and antibiotics (Table 14, p. 145) are sometimes needed. Macular edema is the most common cause for loss of vision, but cataracts, vitreous haze, and glaucoma are also common.

Category A, iritis, inflammation of the iris, accounts for 92% of cases of uveitis. It causes pain, tearing, and photophobia. Signs include miosis (small pupil), perilimbal conjunctival injection (Figs 391–396 and Table 13, p. 144), and anterior chamber flare and cells (Fig. 392).

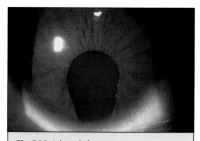

Fig 390 Iris coloboma.

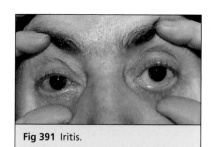

Fig 391 Iritis.

Aqueous

Beam →

Cornea

Iris

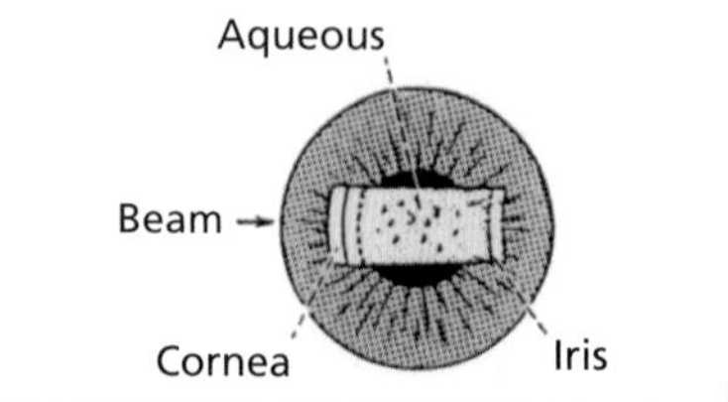

Fig 392 Slit-beam view of flare and cells in anterior chamber.

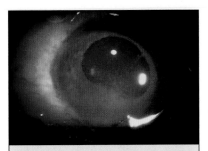

Fig 393 Keratic precipitates (Fig. 395) and posterior synechiae.

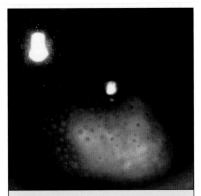

Fig 394 Larger greasy yellowish keratic precipitates called mutton-fat occur in sarcoidosis. Courtesy of University of Iowa, Eyerounds.org.

Flare refers to the beam's milky appearance due to elevated protein. With the slit lamp on high magnification and a short, bright beam shone across the dark pupil, inflammatory cells are graded from trace to very many (4+).

Deposits of inflammatory cells and protein on the corneal endothelium (Figs 393, 394, and 395) are called keratic precipitates (or KPs) and are often a sign that is present for more than a few days. Iritis usually reduces eye pressure due to depressed secretion of aqueous and increased uveoscleral outflow. On the other hand the pressure could become elevated if the drainage from the eye is compromised by uveitic inflammatory cells obstructing the trabecular meshwork or from the side-effect of the corticosteroid used to treat the iritis.

Another complication of iritis is posterior synechiae. These are adhesions between the iris and the lens capsule (Fig. 393). To prevent this, steroids, such as generic topical prednisolone 1% (Pred Forte) or branded diflupred-nate (Durezol) are given to prevent a fibrinous sticky aqueous. Medrysone (HMS 1%), fluorometholone 0.25% (FML Forte), and lotepre-dnol 0.5% (Lotimax) are three examples of

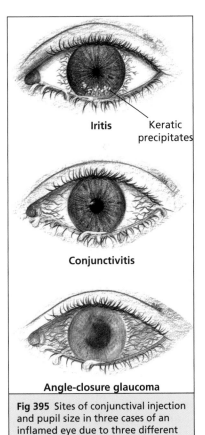

Iritis | Keratic precipitates

Conjunctivitis

Angle-closure glaucoma

Fig 395 Sites of conjunctival injection and pupil size in three cases of an inflamed eye due to three different causes (Figs 305, 363, and 393).

	Iritis	*Conjunctivitis*	*Acute glaucoma* (Fig. 364)
Symptom	Pain, photophobia	Gritty, itching	Pain (often severe), photophobia
Discharge	Tearing	Pus, mucus, or tears	Tearing
Pupil	Miotic	Normal	Mid-dilated
Injection	Limbal	Diffuse	Diffuse and limbal
Cornea	Keratin precipitates	Clear	Steamy cornea
Pressure	Usually low	Normal	Elevated
Anterior chamber	Flare and cells (Figs 382 to 392)	Normal	Shallow

Table 13 Common causes of an injected conjunctiva (Fig. 395).

steroids with less pressure-elevating effects, but are less potent. Frequency and strength of medication depends on the severity of the condition (Table 14, p. 145).

Anti-inflammatories

Corticosteroids have been the mainstay of therapy for non-infectious ocular inflammation since their initial use in the 1950's (Fig. 367 and Table 14, p. 145). They are used to treat autoimmune diseases, uveitis, post-operative inflammation, allergic and infectious conjunctivitis, keratitis, scleritis, episcleritis, and Grave's orbitopathy. They are commonly given by eye drop to treat anterior uveitis. Subconjunctival subtenons or retrobulbar injections are used for severe anterior uveitis, intermediate uveitis, and posterior uveitis. The drug passes easily through the sclera, bypassing the corneal and conjunctival barriers. Chronic, more severe, non-infectious posterior uveitis may be treated with an intravitreal steroid injection or implant, especially if it is chronic causing macular edema. These implants absorb over months. Oral steroids, which have more side effects, may also be tried in resistant cases. Systemic immune-suppressive drugs—most commonly methotrexate—are

Table 14 Ocular Anti-inflammatories (see Fig. 367).

	Brand		Comment
Stronger steroid drops for post-op and uveitis	Durezol	Difluprednate 0.05%	Most potent, but only brand
	Pred Forte (g)	Prednisolone 1%	Generic
	Lotemax	Loteprednol 0.5%	Less pressure elevation (weaker effect)
Weaker steroid drops	Pred Mild	Prednisolone 0.12%	For significant allergy, conjunctivitis, severe dry eye, episcleritis
	Alrex	Loteprednol 0.2%	
	Flarex	Fluorometholone 0.1%	
	FML	Fluorometholone 0.1%	
	FML Forte	Fluorometholone 0.25%	
Steroid ointment and gel	Lotemax SM gel	Loteprednol 0.38%	Longer acting than solutions
	Maxidex ointment	Dexamethasone 0.05%	For eye and skin of lid
Steroid intracanalicular insert	Dextenza	Dexamethasone 0.4 mg.	Eliminates post-op steroid drops
Steroid intraocular injection into anterior chamber	Dexycu	Dexamethasone 9%	Eliminates post-op steroid drops – lasts 30 days
Subtenon, subconjunctival or retrobulbar injection	Kenalog	Triamcinolone	Eliminates post-op steroid drops.
		Dexamethasone	Treat scleritis, uveitis, chalazion
Intravitreous injection (Figs 526 and 527)		Triamcinolone	Lasts for weeks – for macular edema, vitreous
(Figs 529 and 530)		Dexamethasone	
Vitreous implant (Figs 367 and 492)	Retisert	Fluocinolone	Lasts for 30 months } To treat non-infectious
(Fig. 493)	Yutiq 0.18 mg	Fluocinolone	Lasts for 36 months } inflammation affecting posterior
	Ozurdex	Dexamethasone	Lasts up to 6 months } segment of the eye
I.V. Methylprednisolone, then longer-term oral prednisone			For optic neuritis due to giant cell arteritis
Non-steroidal anti-inflammatory	Acular	Ketorolac 0.5%	QID post-op

(Continued)

Table 14 (Continued)

	Brand		Comment
drug (NSAIDS) block	Prolensa	Bromfenac 0.07%	Once a day post-op
prostaglandins	Ilevro	Nepafenac 0.3%	Once a day post-op
Anti-metabolite	Oral	Methotrexate	Immune modulator which is steroid-sparing to suppress posterior non-infectious inflammation
Humira	Subcutaneous injection	Methotrexate and Humira often given by a consulting rheumatologist	For severe, difficult to treat, non-infectious posterior and panuveitis
Doxycycline	Oral	20mg or 100 mg tab. BID	Anti-inflammatory and antibiotic effect for blepharitis and infected chalazions

sometimes substituted for oral steroids, since they are safer for long-term use, especially in children. Humira (adalimumab) subcutaneous injections may also be used as steroid-sparing treatment for noninfectious intermediate, posterior, and panuveitis.

Local side effects of corticosteroids include cataracts, glaucoma (Fig. 367), and activation of herpes keratitis (Fig. 258). Systemic side effects include reduced immunity, osteoporosis, and exacerbation of diabetes or gastric ulcers. Topical NSAID drops, such as generic ketorolac 0.5% (Acular), or branded Ilevro or Prolensa are less effective and may be used in addition to the steroid or as a stand-alone treatment, especially in glaucoma patients, since they don't elevate eye pressure. Irreversible glaucoma may occur in 3% of patients treated with steroids.

Cycloplegics—Table 15, p. 147—such as cyclopentolate 1% or longer-acting atropine 1%, are instilled to keep the pupil dilated thereby minimizing the chance of posterior synechiae (Fig. 393) and also to relieve pain and photophobia due to ciliary muscle spasm.

Iritis is caused most often by intraocular surgery, blunt ocular trauma, corneal ulcers, or abrasions, and foreign bodies. Human leukocyte antigen (HLA-B27) is found in 2–9% of

Table 15 Topical Anticholinergics.

Anticholinergic	Action time	Primary use
Atropine 0.5–1%	±2 weeks	Prolonged or severe anterior uveitis
Scopolamine 0.25% (hyoscine 0.25%)	±4 days	Alternative when allergic to atropine
Homatropine 2–5%	±2 days	Anterior uveitis
Cyclopentolate (Cyclogyl) 1–2%	±1 day	Cycloplegic retinoscopy; rapid onset (30 minutes)
Tropicamide (Mydriacyl) 0.5%	±6 hours	Often used with phenylephrine 2.5% or 10% for pupil dilation

normal persons. Of this small group of individuals possessing the HLA-B27 antigen, 20% are predisposed to autoimmune disorders. Iritis may be associated with the following five HLA-B27-positive autoimmune diseases:

1 ankylosing spondylitis (mostly males with arthritis of the lower spine, of whom 95% are HLA-B27-positive).
2 juvenile idiopathic arthritis, which is typically bilateral and could be asymptomatic. There is an increased risk of cataract formation due to uveitis and use of corticosteroids.
3 reactive arthritis (formerly Reiter's syndrome), in males with urethritis and conjunctivitis.
4 inflammatory bowel disease.
5 psoriatic arthritis.

Causes that are not related to HLA-B27 levels are toxoplasmosis, sarcoidosis, Lyme disease, influenza, lymphoma, AIDS, herpes simplex and zoster (shingles), and Behcet's disease (ulcers in the mouth and genitals) (Fig. 396). There are other even rarer etiologies. Therefore, careful clinical judgment is needed in determining the timing and extent of the workup, taking into consideration cost, severity, chronicity, and associated medical history (see Table 16, p. 148).

Patients with juvenile idiopathic arthritis and chronic iritis often develop a band of calcification in Bowman's membrane known as band keratopathy (Fig. 397). It may be removed by using a technique called chelation in which

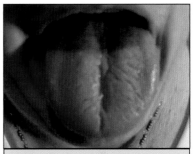

Fig 396 Patient with Behcet's disease with ulcers and fissures on her tongue. She complained of constant burning in mouth.

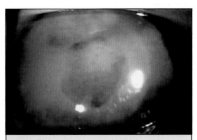

Fig 397 Band keratopathy with calcium deposits in Bauman's membrane in central cornea due to sarcoidosis. Other causes include hypercalcemia, phthisis (Fig. 230), trauma, superficial keratitis, and uveitis.

Table 16 Causes of Uveitis.

A workup for uveitis is necessary when it is prolonged, recurrent, or severe. The following screening tests for most common causes should be considered depending on the geographic location, age of patient, and other signs and symptoms. An extensive workup could be postponed if there are signs of "common cold," influenza, or a history of herpes simplex shingles (herpes zoster), intraocular surgery, corneal inflammation, and ocular trauma. A copy of this table could be sent to their primary care physician, with your suggestions for workup.

Diagnosis	Major clues	Laboratory evaluation
AIDS (Figs 416-419)	Malaise, weight loss, lymphadenopathy, and signs of infection, especially toxoplasmosis, cytomegalovirus, and herpes simplex	HIV-1, HIV-2, antibody screen
Ankylosing spondylitis	Often males with lower back pain	HLA-B27, sacroiliac and lumbar spinal X-ray
Anterior uveitis (HLA-B27+)	Associated with ankylosing spondylitis, inflammatory bowel disease, psoriasis, reactive arthritis (formerly Reiter's syndrome), juvenile idiopathic arthritis	HLA-B27
Behcet's disease	Young adults with mouth and genital ulcers, and skin lesions	HLA-B51
Coccidioidomycosis	Chorioretinitis, fever, cough; endemic along coast of California, Mexico, and South America	Serum antibodies
Cytomegalovirus	Most commonly in AIDS; severe retinitis (Fig. 534)	CMV antibody titer
Presumed histoplasmosis (fungus)	Multiple, small, chorioretinal lesions (histo spots) (Fig. 409) linked to bird droppings along the Ohio and Mississippi river valleys 350,000 cases/year in the USA	Histoplasmin skin test
Juvenile idiopathic arthritis	Children, fever with hepatosplenomegaly (Still's disease)	+ANA 75% of time
Lyme disease	Tick bite, skin rash, arthropathy, neurologic symptoms, mostly in New England and mid-Atlantic states	Serum anti-*Borrelia burgdorferi* antibodies
Lymphoma	Vitritis and anterior uveitis	MRI of brain (Fig. 120), lumbar puncture, and/or vitreous cytology
Multiple sclerosis	Intermediate uveitis, neurologic symptoms, especially optic neuritis	MRI of brain
Polyarteritis nodosa	Systemic necrotizing vasculitis causing fatigue, myalgia, weight loss, nephritis, fever, arthralgia, iritis, keratitis, scleritis	↑ ESR, biopsy of artery confirms diagnosis, ↑ blood urea nitrogen
Reactive arthritis (formerly Reiter's syndrome)	Iridocyclitis, urethritis, arthritis	75% (+) HLA-B27, elevated ESR, ANA

(Continued)

Table 16 (Continued)

Rheumatoid arthritis	Joint pain, anemia	Rheumatoid factor +85% of time (elevated ESR)
Sarcoidosis (Figs 398-407)	Breathing disorder most common, panuveitis, lymph node enlargement	Chest X-ray, biopsy of skin, conjunctiva, lymph node, or lacrimal gland; serum ACE
Sjögren's syndrome	Mainly women, dry eye and mouth, arthritis	Anti-SSA/Ro and anti-SSB, subtypes of ANA
Syphilis (Figs 411-415)	Retinitis, choroiditis, multitude of systemic symptoms	RPR or VDRL
Systemic lupus erythematosus (Fig. 4)	90% women, macular rash, oral and nasal ulcers, discoid lupus, arthritis, pleurisy, pericarditis	ANA is + in 95% of SLE
Toxoplasmosis (Fig. 408) (intracellular protozoa)	Very common; anterior and posterior uveitis; often in AIDS	Serum anti-*Toxoplasma gondii* antibodies: 23% of USA population have + antibody
Toxocariasis (roundworm)	Posterior uveitis in toddlers with exposure to dog or cat	6% of USA population positive for serum ELISA antibodies to *Toxocara*; eosinophilia
Tuberculosis (infects 20–43% of world population)	Cough, fever, weight loss, malaise, and sweats	Chest X-ray, PPD skin test + in 4% of USA. Mycobacteria in sputum
Granulomatosis and polyangiitis (formerly Wegener granulomatosis)	Autoimmune uveitis and retinitis; often involves upper and lower respiratory tracts, but also kidneys and CNS; orbital pseudotumor (Fig. 228) occurs in 45% of patients	Chest X-ray shows cavitary lesions and pneumonitis; biopsy any involved tissue, antineutrophil cytoplasmic antibody positive in only 40%

ACE, angiotensin converting enzyme; ANA, antinuclear antibody; anti-SSA, SSB, types A and B anti-Sjögren's syndrome antinuclear antibodies; ESR, erythrocyte sedimentation rate; PPD, purified protein derivative skin test; RPR, rapid plasma reagin; VDRL, Venereal Disease Research Laboratory.

the calcium is dissolved by applying ethylene-diaminetetraacetic acid (EDTA) to the cornea. Laser keratectomy may also be used.

Category B Intermediate uveitis includes inflammation of the ciliary body (cyclitis), pars plana, and vitreous. The cyclitis often causes pain in and around the eye, and 80% of the time one sees cells in the vitreous. Multiple sclerosis and sarcoidosis (Figs 398–407) are most common causes. Cigarette smoking, trauma, neoplasm, and infections such as Lyme disease and syphilis should be considered. Often no cause is found. It causes pain and decreased eye pressure. Vitreous cells and/or macular edema result in loss of vision. It often requires systemic treatment.

Sarcoidosis

Sarcoidosis is a systemic disease of unknown etiology characterized in 75% of patients by granulomatous inflammation of the lung (Fig. 398). It also affects skin (Fig. 406), peripheral nerves, liver, kidney, and other tissues. The main ocular finding is iritis often associated with large, greasy (mutton-fat) keratic precipitates (Fig. 399). Lacrimal gland granulomas (Figs 403 and 404), intermediate uveitis, and vasculitis (Fig. 407) occur less frequently. It is usually treated with local or systemic corticosteroids.

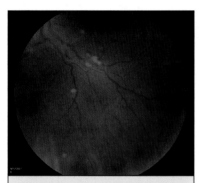

Fig 400 Sarcoidosis with intermediate uveitis and "snowballs" of inflammatory cells in the peripheral vitreous. *Source*: Courtesy of Julia Monsonego, CRA, Wills Eye Hospital.

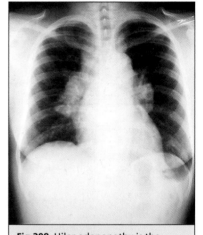

Fig 398 Hilar adenopathy is the number one sign of sarcoidosis occurring in 75% of cases.

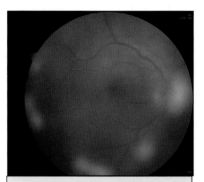

Fig 401 Intermediate uveitis (pars planitis) with snowballing of inflammatory cells on the pars plana. *Source*: Courtesy of Careen Lowder, MD, Cole Eye Institute.

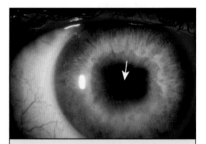

Fig 399 Iritis occurs in 25% of patients with sarcoidosis and is the number one ocular finding. Above are large smooth (mutton-fat) keratic precipitates and an irregular pupil due to posterior synechiae. *Source*: Courtesy of Aman K. Farr, MD, and *Arch. Ophthalmol.*, May 2000, Vol. 118, Nos 1–6, p. 729. Copyright 2000, American Medical Association. All rights reserved.

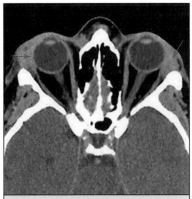

Fig 402 CT scan of sarcoidosis with bilaterally enlarged lacrimal glands (↑). This patient also had lung, skin, conjunctiva, and kidney involvement.

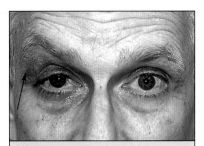

Fig 403 Sarcoidosis with visibly enlarged right lacrimal gland (↑). Notice elevated right brow and ptosis.

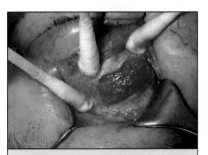

Fig 404 A lacrimal gland biopsy often helps confirm the diagnosis of sarcoidosis.

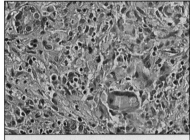

Fig 405 Light photomicrograph of lacrimal gland infiltrated with non-caseating granuloma in sarcoidosis.

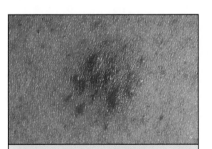

Fig 406 Tender erythematous subcutaneous sarcoid nodule. *Source*: Courtesy of Dr John Woogend and *Arch. Ophthalmol.*, May 2007, Vol. 125, pp. 707–709. Copyright 2007, American Medical Association. All rights reserved.

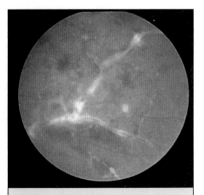

Fig 407 Sarcoidosis with vasculitis causing "candle-wax" drippings on vessel. *Source*: Courtesy of Joseph Walsh, MD.

Category C, Choroiditis, is characterized by white exudates extending onto the retina (Fig. 408A). It is sometimes obscured from view by cells in the vitreous. It leads to chorioretinal atrophy with pigment mottling (Fig. 408B) and macular edema. Often no cause is found, but the following etiologies should be considered.

Causes of choroiditis

1 Bacterial: syphilis (Figs 411–415); tuberculosis is the biggest infectious disease killer worldwide and claims 1.5 million lives each year. It spreads through the air and is consequently increasing due to indoor quarantine during the COVID-19 pandemic.
2 Viral: herpes simplex, cytomegalovirus in 25% of AIDS patients (Figs 416–419 and 534).
3 Fungal: histoplasmosis (Figs 409 and 524), candidiasis.
4 Parasitic: *Toxoplasma* (Fig. 408), *Toxocara* (Fig. 410).
5 Immunosuppression: AIDS predisposes to several of the above.
6 Behcet's disease (mouth and genital ulcers with vasculitis and dermatitis) (Fig. 396).
7 Sympathetic ophthalmia (Figs 420–426)

Choroiditis often requires subconjunctival intravitreal or systemic steroids, especially

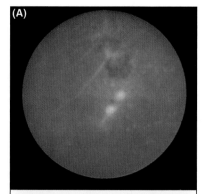
(A)

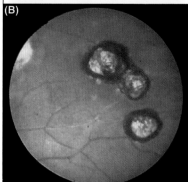
(B)

Fig 408 (A) *Toxoplasma gondii* is an intracellular parasite. It is the most common cause of infectious chorioretinitis. Up to 25% of lamb and pork in the USA harbor cysts. One quarter of people are seropositive. It is spread by congenital or oral transmission. Most common treatment is oral pyrethamine and sulfadiazine combined with systemic corticosteroid. Active lesion appears as a "headlight in a fog" due to cells in the overlying vitreous. (B) Old scar showing hyperpigmentation with white sclera showing through atrophic retina and choroid.

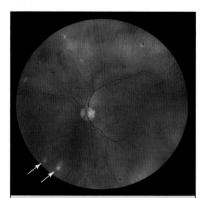

Fig 409 Histoplasmosis with multiple punched out chorioretinitic lesions called "histo spots." *Source:* Courtesy of Alexis Smith, CRT, OCT-T, Kellogg Eye Center, Michigan.

when it threatens the macula, optic nerve, or the associated vitritis reduces vision or is a potential source of membrane formation.

Parasitic worms, sometimes referred to as microfilaria, may infect humans (Fig. 410). *Toxocara canis* and *Toxocara cati* are microfilaria transmitted by the oral ingestion of ova. Toddlers may ingest them by playing on the ground where animals have defecated and adults may ingest them by eating unwashed vegetables.

Don't confuse the *Toxocara* nematode, which is an extracellular parasite, with the other similar-sounding parasite, *Toxoplasma*, which lives inside the cell. However, what toxocariasis and toxoplasmosis have in common is that both may cause severe intraocular inflammation.

Onchocerca volvulus, found 95% of the time in Africa, afflicts people living along riverbanks. It is responsible for 270,000 cases of blindness caused by scarring of the cornea, optic neuritis, and chorioretinitis. The disease is often called "river blindness." Another African worm—*Loa loa*—can migrate to the lids and conjunctiva where it can live for up to 17 years and cause inflammation.

Syphilis

This infectious disease (Figs 411–415), caused by *Treponema pallidum*, is usually transmitted through sexual contact. It can infect any organ of the body. Ocular involvement usually includes the uvea, resulting in iritis, cyclitis, and chorioretinitis. Neurosyphilis could involve all the cranial nerves and cause the pupillary response called the Argyll Robertson pupil. Here, the pupils may be irregularly constricted with decreased or absent response to light, but a normal near reflex. The pupil dilates poorly with mydriatics. Sadly, the incidence of syphilis increased almost every year between 2000 and 2018.

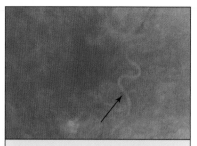

Fig 410 Unknown southeastern US subretinal nematode (↑) causing neuroretinitis. *Source*: Courtesy of J. Donald M. Gass, MD, and *Arch. Ophthalmol.*, Nov. 1983, Vol. 101, No. 3, pp. 1689–1697. Copyright 1983, American Medical Association. All rights reserved.

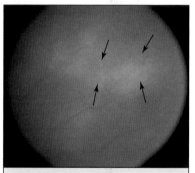

Fig 411 Syphilitic, yellow, flat chorioretinal lesions. *Source:* Courtesy of Thomas R. Friberg, MD, and *Arch. Ophthalmol.*, Nov. 1989, Vol. 107, pp. 1571–1572. Copyright 1989, American Medical Association. All rights reserved.

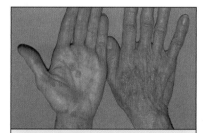

Fig 412 Maculopapular syphilitic eruption involving palms.

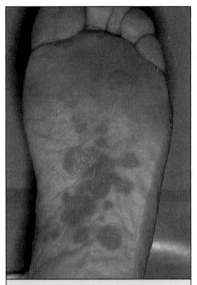

Fig 413 Maculopapular syphilitic eruption involving soles.

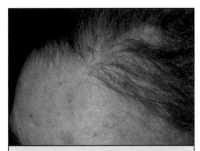

Fig 414 Syphilitic zones of alopecia prompted patient to wear a wig.

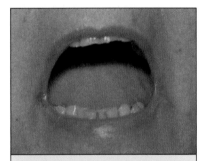

Fig 415 Syphilitic painless mucous membrane ulcers occurred at the corners of patient's mouth.

Human immunodeficiency virus (HIV)

This retrovirus invades and inactivates the CD4+ T-lymphocytes of the immune system. Fortunately, the incidence has decreased in recent years. In 2019, 1.7 million US citizens and 38 million people worldwide became infected. Initially, it may cause weight loss, headache, malaise, fever, chills, and lymphadenopathy, with retinopathy (Figs 418, 419, and 534) in the later stages of AIDS. When the CD4+ T-cells drop from the normal of 500–1500 cells/mm^3 to less than 200 cells/mm^3, the acquired immune deficiency syndrome (AIDS) begins. AIDS occurs in 38.3% of those infected with HIV within a year of diagnosis and 45% within 3 years. Up to 90% of adults in the USA harbor herpes simplex virus, 40–80% have cytomegalovirus (CMV), and 25% have antibodies to *Toxoplasma gondii* (Figs 408A and B). These three opportunistic organisms are among the most common to become virulent in immunocompromised patients with AIDS.

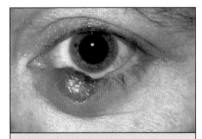

Fig 416 Kaposi's sarcoma of skin in AIDS due to the opportunistic infection by herpesvirus 8. *Source*: Courtesy of Jerry Shields, MD.

If the CD4+ T-cell count is >200 cells/mm³ with no ocular disease, a yearly eye exam is adequate; otherwise, the patient is at increased risk from opportunistic infection and should be examined every 4 months. Highly active antiretroviral therapy (HAART) a "cocktail" of medication should be started at the detection of HIV virus. It is not a cure, but slows the progression. Without treatment, nearly every patient with HIV will get AIDS. Medications or the disease could cause uveitis, vitritis, epiretinal membranes, or acute retinal necrosis that could lead to retinal detachment. HAART therapy, together with Vitrasert (ganciclovir) intravitreal implants, has resulted in a reduction in both HIV- and CMV-associated mortality and a 90% reduction in retinitis complications in the USA. Kaposi's sarcoma (Figs 416 and 417) is the malignancy seen most often in AIDS. There is a non-tender purple nodule on the skin or conjunctiva. Rx: radiation or excision. In 2018, 37,968 people in the USA received a diagnosis of HIV resulting in 1.2 million living with this disease. It caused 15,820 deaths in that year.

Sympathetic ophthalmia

This is a rare condition. It refers to a traumatic or surgical injury (Figs 420–423) to the uvea of one eye resulting in a chronic, immune panuveitis involving both eyes. It may occur after 1:300 eye injuries or 1:1000 intraocular surgeries. A penetrating injury through the corneoscleral wall is referred to as an open-globe injury (Figs 419–422). Handle the eye with minimal probing. Place the patient at rest with bilateral shields that exert no pressure and start intravenous broad-spectrum antibiotics. Call the eye surgeon immediately. If the uvea or retina are extruded from the eye and it cannot be repaired, the eye is removed (enucleated) (Figs 423–426). A spherical prosthesis made of acrylic, silicone (Fig. 424), polymethylmethacrylate, or hydroxyapatite (Fig. 425). A removable scleral prosthesis fit by an ocularist is painted to match the other eye and is placed on the conjunctiva. Enucleation should be performed within 10 days of the

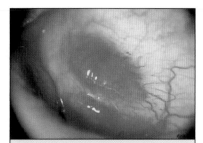

Fig 417 Kaposi's sarcoma of conjunctiva. *Source:* Courtesy of Jerry Shields, MD.

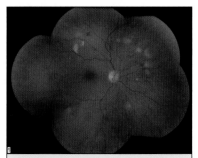

Fig 418 AIDS retinopathy with cotton-wool spots and intraretinal hemorrhages occurs in 50% of patients with AIDS. There is no treatment. *Source:* Courtesy of Julia Monsonego, CRA Wills Eye Hospital.

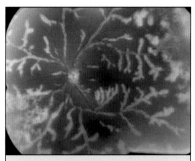

Fig 419 Cytomegalovirus (CMV) is the most frequent opportunistic infection in patients with AIDS. Retinitis is a significant risk factor for mortality. This case shows frosted retinal angiitis. *Source:* Courtesy of Harry Flynn, MD, and *Retinal Physician*, Oct. 2010, Vol. 7, No. 8, p. 67.

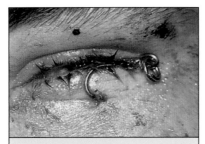

Fig 420 Fishhook in eye.

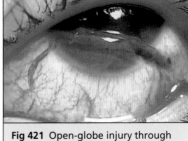

Fig 421 Open-globe injury through corneoscleral wall with prolapse of iris and ciliary body.

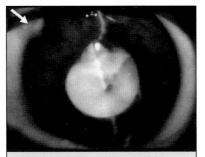

Fig 422 Penetrating injury through iris and lens capsule causing a cataract which must be removed due to damage from leakage of contents.

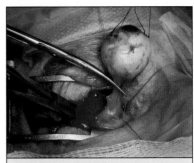

Fig 423 Enucleation: the eye is removed by first exposing and then severing the insertions of the six extraocular muscles. Then the optic nerve is cut as shown above. An eye may be removed when it is blind, painful, cosmetically unappealing, or harbors a tumor and to avoid a sympathetic immune response in the other eye. *Source*: Courtesy of Jeffrey Nerad, MD.

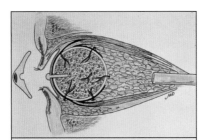

Fig 425 Porous hydroxyapatite implant allows ingrowth of blood vessels to prevent migration or extrusion. Muscles may be sutured to surface polymer coating the implant that months later absorbs after the muscles adhere to provide more normal movement. *Source*: Courtesy of Integrated Orbital Implants, Inc.

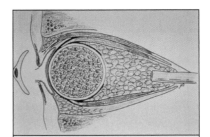

Fig 424 Silicone orbital implant with scleral prosthesis. *Source*: Courtesy of Integrated Orbital Implants, Inc.

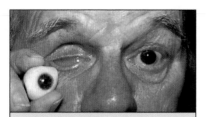

Fig 426 Enucleated socket with scleral prosthesis.

injury to prevent sympathetic ophthalmia. If the rare occurrence of sympathetic ophthalmia does occur, corticosteroids and immunomodulatory (Table 14, p. 145) therapy may be required for many years and possibly decades.

A blind, severely atrophic anatomically disfigured eye called phthisis bulbi (Fig. 230) may also be removed for cosmetic reasons, to relieve pain, or if it harbors a malignancy or severe infection unresponsive to treatment.

Chapter 9
Cataracts

Cataracts, (the white-water rapids of the Nile), prevented potential invasions, but also kept the Egyptians from going very far.

A *cataract* is a cloudy lens that blocks and scatters the light passing through it, and it occurs in everyone to some degree with aging. It should be suspected especially when elderly patients complain of blurry vision and glare. One sign is that it causes a hazy view of the retina with an ophthalmoscope. The lens consists of an outside capsule surrounding a soft cortical substance and a hard inner nucleus (Fig. 427). The diagnosis is confirmed with a slit lamp and described in the following ways.

1 By etiology: it is usually due to aging, but may be congenital or brought on by radiation, ultraviolet light, diabetes, trauma (perforation of capsule) (see Fig. 422), or steroids. Steroid used to treat chronic iritis in juvenile idiopathic arthritis almost always causes cataracts. There is twice the incidence in cigarette smokers. Juvenile cataracts are rare. Fifty eight percent are idiopathic, 13% are traumatic, and 12% are inherited. There are over 100 congenital syndromes associated with cataracts, most notably, Down's and Marfan's syndromes. All children should have a full eye exam before age 4–5 to uncover cataracts, and, more commonly, amblyopia. Children with rare syndromes should be checked even earlier.

2 By location in lens: cortex (Fig. 428), nucleus, or posterior subcapsule (often due to steroids; Fig. 429).

3 By color or pattern: the infantile inherited type is located in or around the nucleus, and is often non-progressive. A mature, dark brown lens is often hard and difficult to emulsify (Fig. 431) during cataract surgery.

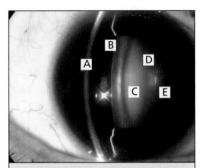

Fig 427 Slit lamp view of lens: A, cornea; B, anterior capsule; C, nucleus; D, posterior cortex; E, posterior capsule. *Source*: Courtesy of Takashi Fujkado, MD.

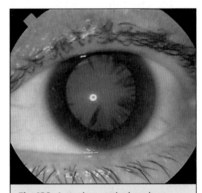

Fig 428 Anterior cortical spokes.

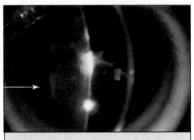

Fig 429 Posterior subcapsular cataract.

Manual for Eye Examination and Diagnosis, Tenth Edition. Mark W. Leitman.

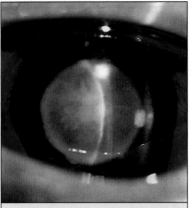

Fig 430 Congenital (zonular) cataract surrounded by clear cortex.

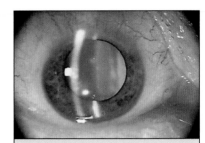

Fig 431 Brunescent (brown) cataract.

A cataract raises two questions. Is it responsible for the decreased vision? Is it ripe? Ripe is the layperson's term for whether surgery is indicated. In most cases, a surgeon waits for a reduction in vision to 20/40 or worse. It is the number one surgery in the USA and worldwide. Indications vary with the patient's needs. Surgery is usually elective except in the rare cases of a mature lens that might rupture (Figs 422, 430, and 432), or with a dislocated lens in imminent danger of dropping into the vitreous or anterior chamber. Lens dislocation (Figs 432 and 433) is due to a rupture of the zonules. It may occur with trauma (Fig. 234) or may be associated with pseudoexfoliation (Fig. 368), Marfan's disease, homocystinuria, or syphilis.

The surgery is performed as an outpatient procedure using local anesthesia. Xylocaine may be injected into the orbit (Fig. 236) or into the anterior chamber. The 10-mm lens may be removed through a 3-mm incision by breaking it up with a phacoemulsifier. The cornea is entered with a blade or laser, making a tunnel incision to minimize chance of leakage and the need for sutures (Fig. 434). If testing of the wound shows leakage, sutures may be used. Iris may prolapse into gaping wound (Fig. 435) and hypotony may cause folds in the cornea called stria (Fig. 267), choroidal effusions (Fig. 351) and macular edema (Fig. 350).

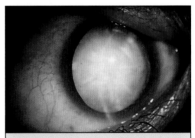

Fig 432 Mature lens dislocated into the anterior chamber, obscuring pupil and iris.

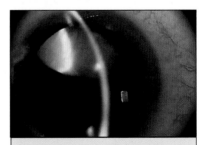

Fig 433 Superiorly dislocated lens.

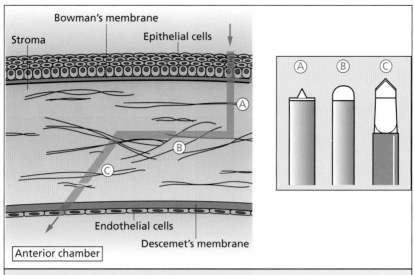

Fig 434 A three-plane corneal incision for entering the eye during cataract surgery. Blade A is guarded to create a uniform mid-depth incision approximately 3–6 mm in length. Blade B is crescent shaped for a 4-mm dissection of corneal lamellae. A downward motion with the keratome (blade C) enters the anterior chamber. A watertight closure is critical to prevent fluid egress or ingress as the incision is getting smaller. There is an increase in preference for one- or two-plane incisions.

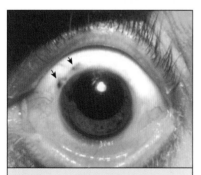

Fig 435 Iris prolapse into gaping wound causing superiorly peaked pupil. *Source*: Courtesy of Eyerounds. org., Univ. of Iowa.

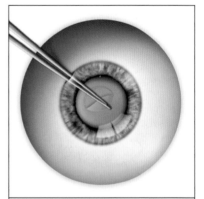

Fig 436 Laser or manual continuous tear capsulotomy (capsulorrhexis). Trypan blue dye may be used to stain this capsule when it is difficult to see.

The anterior lens capsule is then removed (Fig. 436). The majority of the time a laser or continuous tear capsulotomy, called capsulorrhexis, is used, or needle punctures to complete an aborted attempt (Fig. 437) at a 360° tear. The hard nucleus is rarely extracted in one piece (Fig. 441). To facilitate removal of the nucleus through a small wound, it is

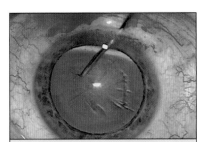

Fig 437 Anterior capsulotomy needle. Punctures of the anterior capsule could be used to complete a less than successful 360° tear. *Source*: Courtesy of Richard Tipperman, MD, and Stephen Lichtenstein, MD.

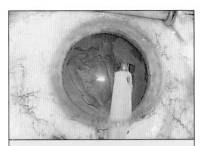

Fig 438 Removal of nucleus by phacoemulsification. *Source*: Courtesy of Richard Tipperman, MD, and Stephen Lichtenstein, MD.

fragmented with a phacoemulsifier, which has a tip that vibrates 40,000 times per second (Fig. 438). (*Phaco-* is a prefix referring to the lens.) Phacoemulsification's disadvantage is that it requires a lot of energy to liquefy a hard nucleus. This could damage the corneal endothelium or the delicate posterior lens capsule, and the risk may be minimized by initially using a laser to partially breakup the hard nucleus (Fig. 447).

A less expensive alternative to phacoemulsification that is sometimes used in the developing world is manual fracture (Figs 439 and 440). An especially black, hard nucleus could also be removed in one piece through a larger incision, since too much phaco energy required could damage the cornea (Fig. 441). After the nucleus is removed by either method, the soft cortex is aspirated (Fig. 442), and the eye is referred to as *aphakic*. A spectacle

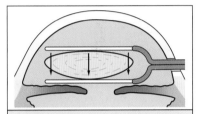

Fig 439 Manual phacofragmentation of nucleus after dislocation into anterior chamber. A platform is placed under the nucleus and a chopper is pushed down to divide it.

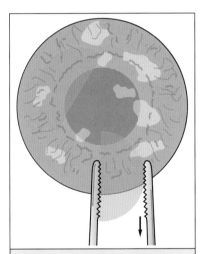

Fig 440 After cracking the hard nucleus, it is removed in two pieces with toothed forceps through a 5 mm wound. Note the white cortex still to be aspirated.

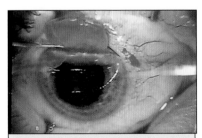

Fig 441 Removal of hard nucleus in one piece. *Source*: Courtesy of Richard Tipperman, MD and Stephen Lichtenstein, MD.

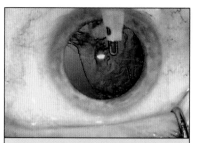

Fig 442 After removing the hard nucleus by any technique, the surrounding cortex is removed with irrigation and aspiration. *Source:* Courtesy of Richard Tipperman, MD, and Stephen Lichtenstein, MD.

lens of about +12.0 D would be required to focus the eye, but it is thick and magnifies the image 33% larger than the normal eye, so that the two eyes cannot fuse. A contact lens that magnifies the image to a lesser degree than a spectacle lens can minimize the problem of image size disparity (aniseikonia) and allow binocular vision. However, contact lenses are impractical with elderly patients. Therefore, an acrylic or silicone lens implant of about +18.0 D is inserted into the eye to restore distance vision and the eye is then referred to as *pseudophakic*. A-scan ultrasound is used to measure the anteroposterior diameter of the eye. This length, together with the corneal curvature, as determined with a keratometer, gives the power of the intraocular lens implant needed. Intraocular lens use is presently being evaluated for its safety profile in infants as young as 7 months of age, but has gained wide acceptance after 2 years of age and is commonplace after age 7. Next, the lens implant is placed behind the iris (Figs 443–445) inside the "bag" of the posterior capsule intentionally left behind. If the posterior capsule or zonules are torn and cannot support the implant, it may be placed behind the iris with sutures to the iris or sclera (Fig. 455) or placed in front of the iris (Fig. 446). This eye is now in focus for distance, but requires a spectacle for near vision.

Multifocal lens implants that focus the eye for near and far are expensive, can cause glare,

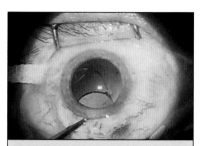

Fig 443 Insertion of rigid lens through a 6-mm incision. *Source:* Courtesy of Richard Tipperman, MD, and Stephen Lichtenstein, MD.

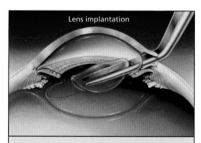

Lens implantation

Fig 444 Foldable implant inserted through a 3.2-mm incision is overwhelmingly preferred.

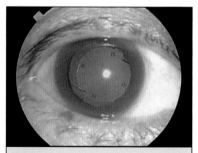

Fig 445 Posterior chamber lens behind iris and in the capsular bag is first choice.

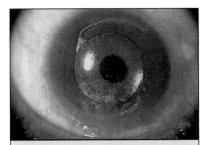

Fig 446 An anterior chamber lens is sometimes used when the posterior capsule or zonules are damaged during surgery and can't support "in the bag" implant. This undesired rupture of the capsule occurs in about 3% of cases.

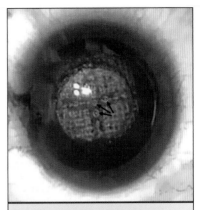

Fig 447 Femtosecond laser-assisted grid fragmentation allows surgeons to soften an especially hard nucleus so that phacoemulsification requires less damaging ultrasound power. *Source:* Courtesy of Richard Witlin, MD.

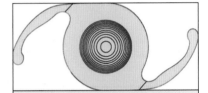

Fig 448 ReSTOR multifocal intraocular lens with 12 concentric steps of focusing power, which allows focus from far to near. It could cause halos and glare, especially at night. Trifocal lenses may be preferred for intermediate rather than very close.

and are only used in about 8% of selected patients so that they might be spectacle-free. One type has alternating rings with different refractive powers (Fig. 448) and the other changes its refractive power by shifting its position with accommodative stimulation to the ciliary body muscle (Fig. 449). In eyes with significant amounts of astigmatism, a more expensive toric implant may be inserted (Fig. 450). Care must be taken in accurately aligning the axis with previously marked locations on the eye and preventing post-operative rotation by gently placing into a capsular bag with intact zonules. Toric multifocal implants are available to correct astigmatism and near vision.

Laser-assisted cataract surgery

In 2018, 10% of cataracts in the USA were removed using laser for part of the procedure. The increased cost and lack of coverage by traditional insurance companies, together with the additional procedure time has made the routine use of femtosecond-laser-assisted cataract extraction quite controversial. Advocates cite four advantages.

1 The laser facilitates capsulotomy (capsulorrhexis). Manually performed continuous circular tear (Fig. 436) capsulotomies are difficult to perform and arguably are not as precise as

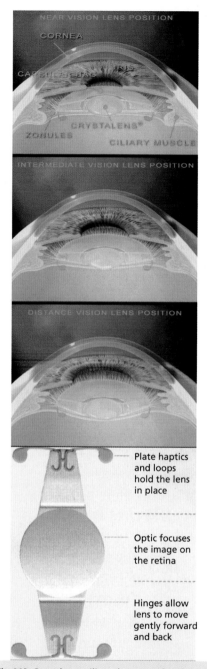

NEAR VISION LENS POSITION
CORNEA
CAPSULE/BAG — IRIS
CRYSTALENS®
ZONULES
CILIARY MUSCLE

INTERMEDIATE VISION LENS POSITION

DISTANCE VISION LENS POSITION

Plate haptics and loops hold the lens in place

Optic focuses the image on the retina

Hinges allow lens to move gently forward and back

Fig 449 Crystalens utilizes the natural action of the ciliary muscle during accommodation to move the optic of the implanted lens forward to focus for near vision. It could minimize glare and halos related to concentric rings in other multifocal implants.

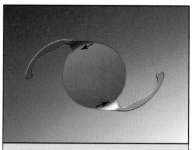

Fig 450 AcrySof IQ Toric intraocular lens. A marker is first used to mark the axis of the astigmatism on the eye. The lens is then inserted so the marks on the lens and eye line up. Techniques require extra care of the capsule to prevent post-op rotation. *Source*: Image courtesy of Alcon Laboratories, Inc.

the laser in reproducing the size and centration of the opening.

2 Emulsification of a hard nucleus with conventional phacofragmentation alone requires extra ultrasound energy. By presoftening and segmenting the nucleus with a laser (Fig. 447), less energy is needed thus protecting intraocular structures, especially the corneal endothelium. The fragments created are of a more predictable size, making aspiration into the phaco tip more predictable.

3 Astigmatism of up to 1.50 D can be corrected during cataract surgery creating one or two partial-thickness arcuate corneal limbus-relaxing incisions (Figs 74–76) to a depth of 90% of corneal thickness. The laser is thought by some to be more precise than a blade. Larger amounts of astigmatism, up to 4.0 diopters, could be eliminated with a more expensive toric implant (Fig. 450).

4 Most cataract surgeries are performed by entering the eye with a blade through a clear peripheral corneal incision of about 3 mm in length. The laser-cut incision may be less prone to wound leaking.

Some complications of cataract surgery

1 The posterior capsule may opacify months to years after cataract extraction and is called a secondary cataract (Fig. 451). It may be opened with an in office YAG laser (Fig. 452).

2 If the zonules tear, the implant could dislocate or decenter (Figs 453–455) in 0.3–3.0% of cases. These implants have to be supported with sutures to the iris or sclera or replaced with a new anterior chamber lens placed in front of the iris (Fig. 446).

3 The corneal endothelium could be damaged, resulting in corneal edema (Figs 248 and 264). It is the most common reason for corneal endothelium transplant surgery, DSEK and DMEK (Figs 272–276).

4 Retinal detachment (Figs 475 and 578) occurs in 1–2% of cataract surgeries, most often in high myopes.

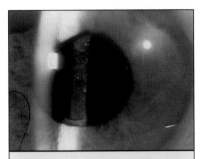

Fig 451 Secondary cataract occurs in 12% of eyes at 1 year and 28% at 5 years after surgery. It is much more common after cataract surgery in children, and many surgeons open this membrane during surgery since there is such a high chance it will cloud over in the short future and having them sit still for a laser procedure in the office is often impossible. *Source*: Courtesy of Richard Tipperman, MD, and Stephen Lichtenstein, MD.

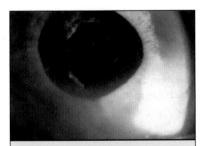

Fig 452 Office-based YAG laser capsulotomy for secondary cataract of posterior capsule. *Source*: Courtesy of Richard Tipperman, MD, and Stephen Lichtenstein, MD.

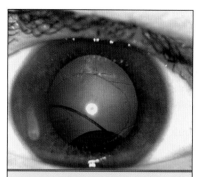

Fig 453 Dislocated intraocular lens due to weakened zonules. *Source*: Courtesy of Elliot Davidoff, MD.

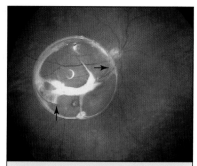

Fig 454 Lens implant (↑ lens haptic) and capsular bag dislocated into the vitreous after traumatic tearing of the zonules. *Source*: Courtesy of S. Parthasarethi, MD, and *Arch. Ophthalmol.*, Sept. 2007, Vol. 125, p. 1240. Copyright 2007, American Medical Association. All rights reserved.

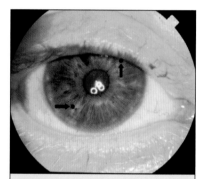

Fig 455 Dislocated posterior chamber lens with haptics sutured to iris. Suturing to sclera instead of the iris results in similar final outcomes, although the latter takes longer to perform.

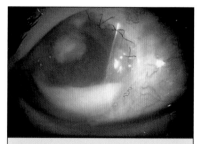

Fig 456 Endophthalmitis with hypopyon following cataract surgery.

5 Infectious endophthalmitis (Figs 456 and 457) is a serious, potentially blinding, complication of cataract surgery or any penetrating intraocular injury. To minimize the chance of this occurring, prophylactic topical pre and post-op broad spectrum antibiotic drops are given and betadine solution is placed on the eye before the start of surgery. If the infection does occur, subconjunctival and intravitreal antibiotics are administered immediately. A vitrectomy is often performed to obtain a sample for culture and to prevent the formation of membranes that cause vitreoretinal traction, which could result in a

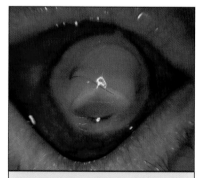

Fig 457 Severe endophthalmitis with visibly dislocated lens implant in anterior chamber. *Source*: Courtesy of Julia Monsonego, CRA, Wills Eye Hospital.

retinal detachment. Fortunately, it only occurs in 1 in 1000 cataract surgeries.

6 Macular edema occurs in 2–60% of cataract surgeries, reducing vision during the post-operative period. It fortunately resolves in almost all cases (see Fig. 523) due to routine use of post-op anti-inflammatory drops and injections.

7 The rarest and worst complication is expulsive hemorrhage. Bleeding into the choroid could propel intraocular contents, including the retina, out of the eye. Be especially cautious with patients on blood thinners or with Sturge-Weber syndrome (Fig. 199).

Chapter 10
The retina and vitreous

Our eyes are always unconsciously scanning the environment. It's called the orienting reflex. The movement stops and the focus intensifies if the stimulus striking the retina signals danger or is a sexual object. Evolution provided us with this survival and reproductive edge. Most other things that are seen are lower priority unless we concentrate on them. Choose wisely!

Retinal anatomy

The retina is the sensory layer of the eye, extending from the optic disk to the ora serrata (Figs 458–461), and has the highest cellular metabolic activity in the body.

Light stimulates 120 million rods, which are mainly located in the peripheral retina. They are very sensitive to small amounts of light critical for night vision. Five million cones, located primarily in the fovea and macula, are responsible for the acute vision needed to read. Both receptor types transmit the message to the ganglion cell on the retinal surface. The long ganglion cell axons exit the eye in the optic nerve, which synapses in the brain

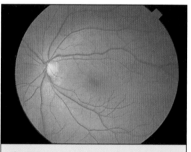

Fig 458 Posterior retinal landmarks.

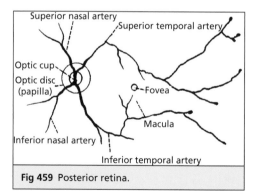

Fig 459 Posterior retina.

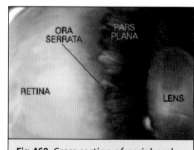

Fig 460 Cross-section of peripheral retina.

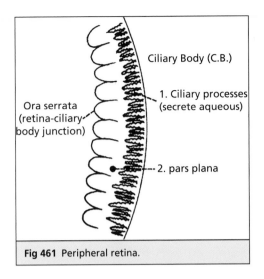

Fig 461 Peripheral retina.

(Fig. 462). Blood is supplied to the inner retina by the central retinal artery (Figs 459 and 507) and the outer retina by the choroidal vessels (Figs 378, 462 and 463).

The macula

The macula is 5 mm in diameter, and its boundaries are defined by the retinal vessels at its margin Fig 459 and cover upper left. In its center is a 1.5-mm avascular pit called the *fovea* (Fig. 463), which produces a light reflex. This reflex decreases with age, and its absence in a young individual with a visual disturbance could indicate macular dysfunction (Compare Figs 490 and 493). When the macula is destroyed, the vision is 20/200 at best.

Optical coherent tomography (OCT) is a noninvasive office device (Figs 338, 339, and 463) that reflects light off the macula at a speed of up to 100,000 scans/s. It may be produced in color or black and white. Resolution to as little as 3 μm has allowed the study of tissues to a cellular level. Low reflectivity appears as black, optically empty space and occurs within a normal vitreous and in cystic areas containing serous fluid and edema. High reflectivity appears white, as with solid membranes (Fig. 463), blood drusen, RPE, choroidal nevi,

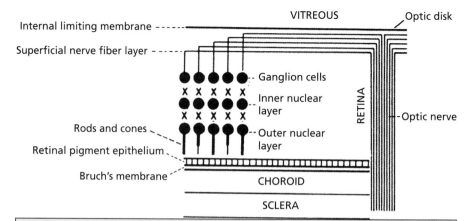

Fig 462 Schematic cross-section of retina. The choroidal blood nourishes the retinal pigment epithelium (RPE) which, in turn, supports the rods and cones. The inner nuclear layer horizontally interconnects the input.

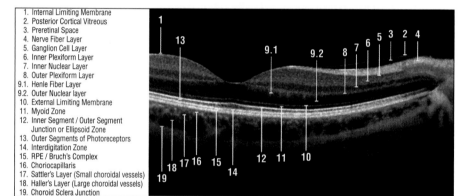

1. Internal Limiting Membrane
2. Posterior Cortical Vitreous
3. Preretinal Space
4. Nerve Fiber Layer
5. Ganglion Cell Layer
6. Inner Plexiform Layer
7. Inner Nuclear Layer
8. Outer Plexiform Layer
9.1. Henle Fiber Layer
9.2. Outer Nuclear layer
10. External Limiting Membrane
11. Myoid Zone
12. Inner Segment / Outer Segment Junction or Ellipsoid Zone
13. Outer Segments of Photoreceptors
14. Interdigitation Zone
15. RPE / Bruch's Complex
16. Choriocapillaris
17. Sattler's Layer (Small choroidal vessels)
18. Haller's Layer (Large choroidal vessels)
19. Choroid Sclera Junction

Fig 463 OCT of normal macula with central foveal pit. Note choroidal-scleral junction (19). The choroidal vessels (16, 17, 18) nourish the retinal pigment epithelium (15) which, in turn, metabolically support the overlying rods and cones that make up the outer nuclear layer. The inner nuclear layer (7) contain the cell bodies that create horizontal synapses interconnecting the stimuli from the rod and cone receptors. The ganglion cells (5) and their axons (4) then exit the eye forming the optic nerve. *Source*: Courtesy of Carl Zeiss, Meditec, Inc.

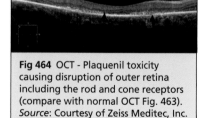

Fig 464 OCT - Plaquenil toxicity causing disruption of outer retina including the rod and cone receptors (compare with normal OCT Fig. 463). *Source*: Courtesy of Zeiss Meditec, Inc.

and scars. It is used to discern fluid within the layers of the retina, especially with respect to macular edema (Figs 490, 499, 500 and 563). It is especially helpful in evaluating the vitreo-retinal interface; macular holes (Figs 568, 569 and 572); age-related macular degeneration (AMD) (Figs 517, 522, 524); and epiretinal membranes (Figs 563 and 572). Optical coherent angiography (OCTA) measures reflections from moving blood and has an advantage over fluorescein angiography because this test is non-invasive and can distinguish capillary structure in the superficial to the deeper retina and choroid (Figs 465, 488B, 505, 506. 507, 508 and 524).

Fundus examination

The fundus refers to the inner part of the eye. It is evaluated with an ophthalmoscope. Eye doctors usually dilate the pupils for this exam. Tropicamide (0.5–1%) (Table 15, p. 147), which relaxes the pupillary sphincter, is preferred because of its quick action (5–10 minutes) and strong effect. Phenylephrine (2.5–10%), which stimulates the dilator muscle, has a weaker effect and takes longer to act (30 minutes). An advantage of phenylephrine is that it does not cause the patient's sight to blur as much and would not be as problematic for them when driving home. Both drugs are often used together when peripheral retinal disease is suspected.

The macula is examined last to minimize miosis and discomfort.

A direct ophthalmoscope (Fig. 466) allows for monocular visualization of the posterior half of the fundus, where most retinal pathology is located. Use a negative lens (red) for myopic eyes and a positive lens (black) for hyperopic eyes. Get as close to the eye as possible and minimize movement by resting the hand that is holding the ophthalmoscope on the patient's cheek, while your other hand lifts the patient's upper lid.

A binocular indirect ophthalmoscope (Fig. 467) consists of a light source worn over

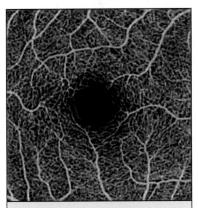

Fig 465 Normal color OCTA of perifoveal retina. Superficial retinal vessels are orange, deep retinal plexus vessels are green. *Source*: Courtesy of Carl Zeiss, Meditec, Inc.

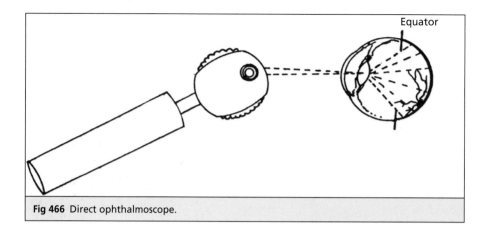

Equator

Fig 466 Direct ophthalmoscope.

the head and a hand-held lens, which allows the retina to be seen in three dimensions, albeit upside down. Retinal holes and detachments at the ora serrata can be viewed by indenting the sclera with a small thimble worn on the index finger (Fig. 461).

A three-mirror contact lens (Figs 468 and 469), used with a slit lamp, gives a detailed stereoscopic view of the entire retina. It is useful in studying subtle changes in each layer of the retina, and to gauge optic cupping. Its disadvantage is the need for anesthetic drops and a gelatinous solution on the eye.

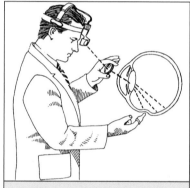

Fig 467 Indirect ophthalmoscope.

Fluorescein angiography

Fluorescein dye is injected intravenously. As it passes through the retinal circulation, fundus photographs are made in a rapid sequence. The dye first appears in arteries in 13 seconds and the veins in 19 seconds. Later images may show leakage and staining of tissues (Figs 477A, 481, 484, 499, and 502). The blood-retinal barrier normally prevents leakage from vessels (Fig. 470). This test is useful for evaluating retinal circulation. It demonstrates rate of flow, leakage from capillaries, staining of tissues, areas of nonperfusion, and neovascularization (Figs 483, 484, 499, 502, and 530). Indications for this invasive test may decrease as improvements continually occur in noninvasive optical coherence angiography.

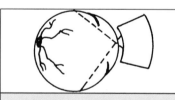

Fig 468 Three-mirror contact lens.

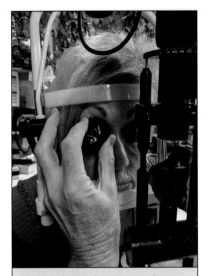

Fig 469 Three mirror contact lens allows detailed three-dimensional visualization of the retina and the angle between the iris and cornea. Note: Image showing use of lens at slit lamp.

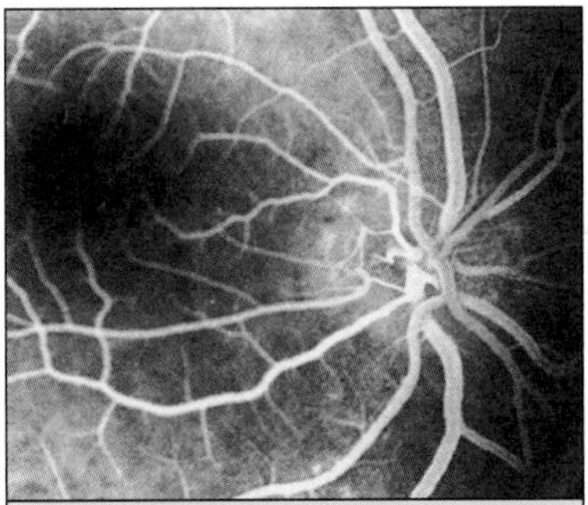

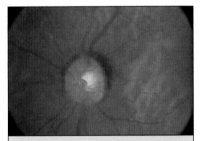

Fig 470 Normal fluorescein angiogram. Retinal vessels terminate at the perifoveal area of the macula. Foveal blood supply comes from underlying choroidal capillaries. The blood-retinal barrier normally prevents leakage from capillaries (see Fig. 502).

The optic disk (papilla)

The optic disk is normally orange–red with a yellow cup at its center. The retinal artery and vein pass through the optic cup and bifurcate on the surface of the disk. Proliferation of the retinal pigment epithelium (RPE) at the disk margin is a normal finding (Fig. 471).

In axial myopia, the eye is increased in length and the retina may be dragged away from the optic disk margin, exposing the sclera. This is called a *myopic conus* or *crescent* (Fig. 472A). In extremely myopic eyes, often greater than 10 D—referred to as *pathologic myopia*—the retina is stretched so thin that it is totally absent in some areas (Fig. 472B).

Another disk variation occurs when the myelin sheath that normally covers the optic nerve extends onto the retina, appearing like white flame-shaped patches obscuring the disk margin. It is benign (Fig. 474). The disk margin may also be obscured by drusen (Fig. 473), which are small, round, translucent bodies made up of hyaline deposits that are often calcified. They occur in 0.3–3.7% of

Fig 471 Normal tigroid (tessellated) fundus with pigment around disk and deeply pigmented choroid.

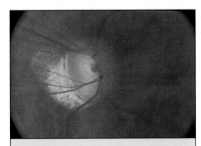

Fig 472A Normal myopic conus (crescent) at disk margin.

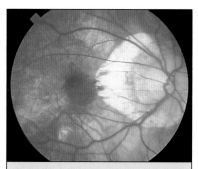

Fig 472B Pathologic myopic happens most often in eyes with more than 10 D of refractive error (Fig. 22). The globe is elongated causing the retina and choroid to be stretched so thin that it causes patchy areas of atrophy exposing the underlying white sclera. *Source*: Courtesy of University of Iowa.

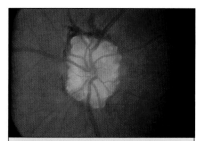

Fig 473 Disk drusen are not related to retinal drusen that occurs in macular degeneration (Figs 516 and 537).

eyes. When superficial, they are easy to identify; but when buried, B-scan ultrasound and CT scanning are needed to reveal calcification (see Figs 479 and 480). Drusen may damage nerve fibers and cause an enlarged blind spot.

Papilledema (choked disk)

Papilledema is swelling of the optic nerve specifically due to elevated intracranial pressure that causes a reduction in the ability of fluid to exit the eye. It is usually bilateral and always serious. The intraocular congestion results in a swollen, elevated optic disk with blurred margins (Figs 475–478). As it progresses, veins become engorged and flame-shaped hemorrhages and cotton-wool spots develop in the peripapillary area (Figs 476, 478).

In 80% of normal eyes, ophthalmoscopic examination reveals subtle pulsations of the retina veins as they exit from the globe at the optic cup. If pulsations are not visible, they can almost always be elicited by exerting slight pressure on the globe (through the lid). In papilledema, one cannot see spontaneous or elicited venous pulsations. Edema of the optic disk may extend to the surrounding retina causing enlargement of the blind spot

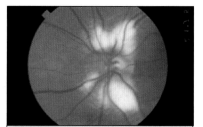

Fig 474 Myelination of the optic nerve. The white myelin sheath covering the optic nerve occasionally extends to the interior of the eye.

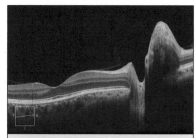

Fig 475 OCT image of papilledema showing elevated disk margin and hyporeflective (black) areas corresponding to edematous fluid in and around the optic disk. Note normal foveal pit temporal to disk. *Source*: Courtesy of Elizabeth Affel, Wills Eye Hospital.

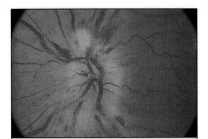

Fig 476 Papilledema with elevated disk, engorged veins, and flame-shaped hemorrhages.

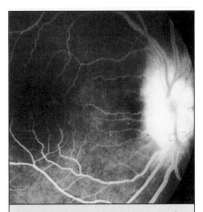

Fig 477A Fluorescein angiogram of papilledema reveals leakage in and around the optic disk.

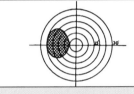

Fig 477B An enlarged blind spot can be plotted most accurately on a tangent screen. Visual field testing of the size of the blind spot and contraction of the peripheral field and OCTs must be monitored closely since this is often the only way to know how the papilledema is being controlled, since serial spinal taps and fluorescein angiograms have more risk.

(Figs 132,134, and 477B). If the fluid extends to the macula, it may reduce central vision (Fig. 478). The central and peripheral vision with the OCT are the safest noninvasive tests to monitor progression or resolution papilledema, since serial spinal taps and fluorescein angiography are more dangerous. Papilledema due to elevated intracranial pressure often causes headache, confusion, nausea, and visual obscurations. Diplopia occurs if the pressure compromises the sixth cranial nerve. Prolonged increased pressure can permanently damage the brain and optic nerve. Common causes are side effects of drugs, such as tetracycline, excessive vitamin A, and retinoids used to treat severe acne and psoriasis. Intracranial brain tumors, hemorrhages, and infections could also elevate intracranial pressure.

Idiopathic intracranial hypertension (pseudotumor cerebri) is a common cause of papilledema. It occurs most often in young overweight women and may be first discovered by noting papilledema during a routine eye exam. Chronic, unrelenting headaches in all patients, but especially these obese women, should remind us to rule out papilledema.

Pseudopapilledema

There are many conditions that can mimic the optic disk changes of papilledema and every clue must be considered.

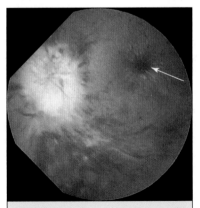

Fig 478 Papilledema with macular star (↑) due to extension of disk edema.

A swollen disk caused by optic neuritis (Fig. 118) is associated with a Marcus Gunn pupil (Fig. 119) and loss of central vision; whereas in early papilledema, the pupil is normal and there is usually no loss of visual acuity unless the disc edema extends to the macula (Fig. 478) or if optic atrophy has already occurred (Fig. 116). Early papilledema may also be difficult to be distinguished from drusen of the disk (Fig. 473) and myelinated nerve fibers (Fig. 474). Both blur the disk margin and cause an enlarged blind spot (Fig. 477B). On fluorescein angiography, however, only papilledema has leakage of dye (Fig. 477A). Like papilledema, central retinal vein occlusion (Fig. 510) may have venous engorgement, flame hemorrhages, a blurred disk margin, and cotton-wool spots. Unlike papilledema in central retinal vein occlusion (Fig. 510), the flame hemorrhages extend out to the peripheral retina and there is more loss of vision. Malignant systemic hypertension (blood pressure 220/120 mmHg) (Table 17, p. 179) also causes a papilledema-like retinal appearance, which is distinguished by measuring blood pressure on all patients with blurry disk margins (Figs 486 and 488A). Orbital diseases decreasing venous outflow from the eye can cause swelling of the disk (Fig. 124). Causes include orbital tumors and infections; idiopathic inflammation of the orbit, also called *orbital pseudotumor* (Figs 226–229B), must be considered. Do not confuse orbital pseudotumor with pseudotumor cerebri (p. 175). In orbital diseases, one looks for localizing signs, such as proptosis. Cavernous sinus disease can also obstruct venous drainage from the orbit (Figs 144–146).

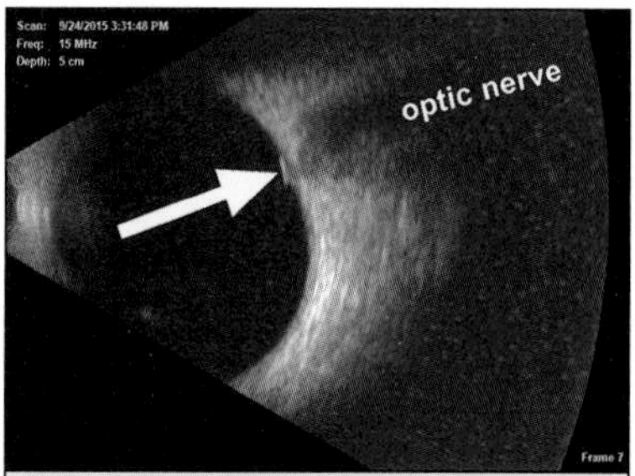

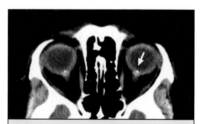

Fig 479 B-Scan ultrasound showing hyperreflective calcification from buried optic disk drusen, which could blur disk margins, confusing it with papilledema. Courtesy of Jonathon Prenner, MD, UMDNJ.

Retinal blood vessels

The retina, brain, and kidney share similar vascular anatomic features and physiologic properties. The retina affords a window into microvascular diseases in these organs. In Alzheimer's disease there may be a loss of retinal blood vessels especially in the perifoveal area. The diagnosis and progression of diabetic kidney disease can be assessed by following the severity of diabetic retinopathy - see cover. Retinal vessel walls are normally

Fig 480 CT scan performed during workup of what was thought to be papilledema instead revealed calcified optic disk drusen. *Source:* Courtesy of Elliot Davidoff, MD, Ohio State Medical School.

transparent. They can be visualized because of the blood they contain. In arteriosclerosis, as the vessel walls become thickened they may develop a silver wire appearance (see cover).

The vessel walls may also whiten when inflamed (Figs 407 and 481) in conditions such as systemic lupus erythematosus, sarcoidosis (Fig. 407), cytomegalovirus infection (Figs 419 and 534), sickle cell disease (Figs 482–484), giant cell arteritis (Fig. 122), toxoplasmosis (Fig. 408), and syphilis. Damaged vessel walls may eventually develop a permanent white sheath and a threadlike lumen (Fig. 496). Loss of blood flow, as occurs in a retinal artery occlusion, diabetes, hypertension, sickle cell disease, and choroiditis may also cause these changes. The resulting ischemia to the ganglion cells may cause cotton-wool spots (cover and Fig. 533).

Abnormal capillaries may grow inside the eye in a misguided response to ischemia most commonly due to diabetic retinopathy. They are due to liberation of vascular endothelial growth factor (VEGF) in response to retinal ischemia. Panretinal photocoagulation (PRP) may be used to destroy large areas of hypoxic retina, thus decreasing the oxygen demand and the secretion of vascular endothelial growth factor (VEGF). A total of 1500 laser burns are usually administered to each eye in two sessions (back cover). In compliant patients—able to return for multiple visits—anti-VEGF injections are an alternative to laser

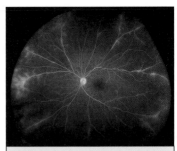

Fig 481 Fluorescein angiogram of vasculitis causing loss of the blood-retina barrier. *Source*: Courtesy of Optos Instruments.

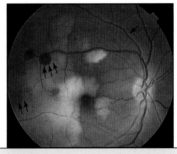

Fig 482 Sickle cell retinopathy with vascular inflammation (↑), pale areas of ischemic retina salmon-patch intraretinal hemorrhages (↑↑), and pre-retinal hemorrhages (↑↑↑). This occurred in a 26-year-old black male presenting to the emergency department with an acute myocardial infarction, renal failure, and cholecystitis.

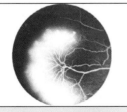

Fig 484 Fluorescein angiogram showing leakage from abnormal new vessels. *Source*: S.B. Cohen et al., *Ophthal. Surg.*, 1986, Vol. 17, No. 2, pp. 110–116. Reprinted with permission from SLACK, Inc.

Fig 483 Sickle cell retinopathy with compensatory neovascularization at edge of infarcted retina with the appearance of a sea fan. *Source*: S. Cohen, et al., Diagnosis and Management of Ocular Complications of Sickle Hemoglobinopathies: Part II. *Ophthalmic Surg Lasers Imaging Retina.*, 1986, Vol. 17, No. 2, pp. 110–116. doi:10.3928/1542-8877-19860201-12. Reprinted with permission from SLACK Incorporated.

PRP for proliferative retinopathy, since the latter significantly reduces peripheral vision.

Introduced in 2006, there currently are four anti-VEGF drugs—ranibizumab (Lucentis), bevacizumab (Avastin), brolucizumab (Beovu), and afibercept (Eylea)—which, when injected into the vitreous, (Figs 526 and 527) cause regression of the abnormal vessels. In 2020, Beavu was reported to cause retinal vasculitis. They are now being used as a first-line treatment of wet macular degeneration and for macular edema due to retinal vein occlusions and diabetic retinopathy. In the USA, 6 million injections were given in 2016, and the indications continue to grow. It is the most common intraocular procedure, even doubling the number of cataract extractions.

Sickle cell hemoglobinopathy leads to red cells taking on a sickle shape in deoxygenated blood (Figs 482–484). Sickle cell trait (HbAS) affects 8% of African Americans, with 0.4% having sickle cell disease (HbSS) and 0.2% having HbSC disease. Retinal neovascularization resembling "sea fans" occur at the edge of infarcted (pale) areas. Confirm with a sickle cell preparation where a deoxygenating agent is added to the patient's blood. It is positive if red blood cells assume a crescent (sickle shape). Treatment with laser or intra-vitreous anti-VEGF is aimed at eliminating these abnormal vessels, which could bleed into vitreous causing fibrotic membranes that could contract and cause retinal detachment (RD) (Figs 485, 504, 562, and 579).

Normal blood pressure (BP) is now considered to be 120/70 or less. Any BP above that is associated with a progressive increase in the risk of heart attack and stroke. The cost, stigma of having a disease, and the side effects of medical treatment usually cause physicians to postpone medicating until BP reaches 140/80 or more. Criteria for treatment varies, but a general rule is to wait for 150/90 in people over age 60 to prevent falls resulting from decreased blood flow to the brain. In diabetics, treatment may be started at levels 10 mm/Hg less than would otherwise be indicated, since both conditions adversely affect the vessels.

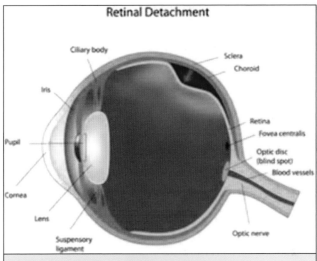

Fig 485 Retinal detachment. *Source*: Alila Medical Media/Shutterstock.com.

Table 17 Scheie classification of hypertensive retinopathy (see Fig. 486).

I	Thinning of retinal arterioles relative to veins	Stages I and II are similar to arteriosclerosis of aging.
II	Obvious arteriolar narrowing with focal areas of attenuation	
III	Stage II, plus cotton-wool spots, exudates, and hemorrhages (Fig. 486)	Stages III and IV are medical emergencies and have strong association with death.
IV	Malignant hypertension, blood pressure 220/120 mmHg Stage III plus swollen optic disk resembling papilledema	

At their junctions, the arteries and veins share a common sheath. As the arteriole wall thickens (arteriosclerosis), it takes on a silvery appearance and causes indentation of the venule, referred to as *A–V nicking* (Fig. 487). This can lead to a retinal vein occlusion.

Retinal vein occlusion (RVO)

Retinal vein occlusions occur in 0.5% of people. The most common cause is aging followed by hypertension. Patients usually present with a sudden, persistent, painless

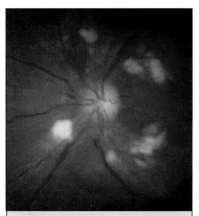

Fig 486 Stage III hypertensive retinopathy with cotton-wool spots, flame-shaped hemorrhages, and arteriolar narrowing (see Table 17, p. 179).

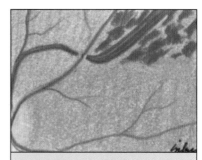

Fig 487 Drawing of branch retinal vein occlusion with flame hemorrhage and a A–V nicking. As the arteriole wall thickens, the A–V crossings change from an acute to a right angle.

decrease in vision. Retinal flame-shaped and dot-and-blot hemorrhages (Figs 487–489, 510 and 512) extend into the periphery and may last for years. Cotton-wool spots and a poorly reactive pupil usually indicate an ischemic retina, which are very ominous. Ischemia is confirmed with fluorescein angiography or OCT angiography (OCTA; Figs 490 and 491). Ischemic cases stimulate secretion of the vascular endothelial growth factor (VEGF) causing new blood vessel growth on the iris, which can bleed and lead to glaucoma (Figs 388 and 389). Not all new vessels are bad. Late-onset, tortuous, retino-choroidal, collateral vessels could develop on the optic disk, and elsewhere in the retina, and are beneficial in helping the obstructed venous blood to exit the eye via the choroidal route (Fig. 489). If macular edema occurs, it is usually treated with intravitreal injections of anti-VEGF or steroid (Figs 526 and 527). Time between injections may vary with responses and is referred to as *treat and extend*. There are corticosteroid intravitreal implants that provide a prolonged slow release (Fig. 492 and Table 13, p.144). Therapy continues until resolution of edema occurs as determined by retinal thickness on OCT (Figs 490 and 493) and return of visual acuity. Treatment should also address the frequently associated risk factors

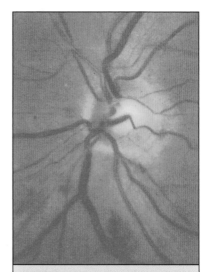

Fig 488A Arteriosclerosis with partial vein occlusion causing an engorged vein inferiorly and a secondary flame hemorrhage. "Silver wire" changes are noted at the superior disk margin.

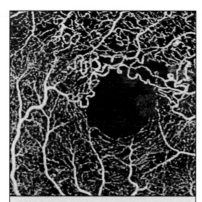

Fig 488B OCT-A of partial vein occlusion with dilated tortuous veins and capillaries. *Source*: Courtesy of Carl Zeiss Meditec, Inc.

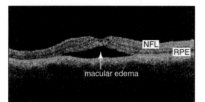

Fig 490 Colored OCT of macular edema after retinal vein occlusion causing thickening of the retina with loss of foveal pit. Measurement of decreasing retinal thickness from edema, together with improvement of vision is used to monitor the response to treatment. Edema also commonly occurs in diabetic retinopathy, wet age-related macular degeneration and in post-op cataract surgery (Figs 522 and 523). RPE (retinal pigment epithelium); NFL (nerve fiber layer).

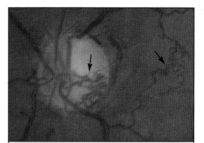

Fig 489 Central retinal vein occlusion 3 months after occurrence. Compensatory collateral curlicue vessels on the disk and retina (↑) help venous blood exit the eye. They do not bleed or leak fluorescein, unlike the pathologic neovascularization that occurs in macular degeneration, and diabetes. *Source*: Courtesy of Julia Monsonego, CRA, Wills Eye Hospital.

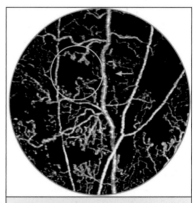

Fig 491 OCT A of branch retinal vein occlusion with tortuous and engorged capillaries and adjacent ischemic area of nonperfusion. *Source*: Courtesy of Carl Zeiss Meditec, Inc.

such as hypertension, dyslipidemia, diabetes, and hypercoagulability of the blood.

Retinal artery occlusion

Retinal artery occlusion (Figs 494–496) causes sudden, painless, loss of vision. Carotid artery plaques (Figs 81, 143, and 585) or heart disease such as arrhythmias, endocarditis (Fig. 528), or valve abnormalities may liberate fine platelets or larger cholesterol emboli (Hollenhorst plaque (Fig. 494)), which often lodge in arterial bifurcations. Sludging of blood flow gives a

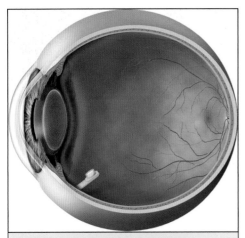

Fig 492 Intravitreal steroidal implants last longer than injection and is considered for chronic macular edema, but requires closer monitoring of eye pressure which could become elevated. *Source*: JirehDesign.com.

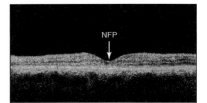

Fig 493 OCT of resolved macular edema from retinal vein occlusion after intravitreal triamcinolone injection. Vision improved from 20/400 to 20/30. NFP, normal foveal pit. *Source*: Courtesy of Jennifer Hancock.

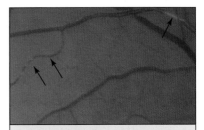

Fig 495 Branch retinal artery occlusion with embolus (↑) and sludging of blood (box-car effect, ↑↑) due to decreased flow. *Source*: Courtesy of Julia Monsonego, CRA, Wills Eye Hospital.

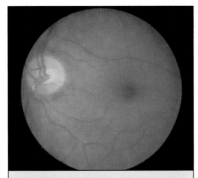

Fig 494 Retinal artery occlusion with a cholesterol Hollenhorst plaque on the disk and a cherry-red spot in the fovea where choroidal blood is seen outlined by a pale, swollen ischemic macula. Most emboli are from the carotid artery. (Figs 81,143 and 584–586).

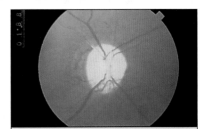

Fig 496 Late-stage retinal artery occlusion with pale disc due to optic atrophy and arteries that are thread-like and sheathed.

box-car appearance (Fig. 495). Some irreparable loss of vision usually occurs within 1 hour, and the loss is almost impossible to reverse after 4–12 hours. Eventually, optic atrophy results (Fig. 496). Any ocular treatment is of questionable value. You could have the patient breathe into a paper bag to elevate CO_2, which dilates the artery; or lower the eye pressure with oral or topical medications. Gently massaging the eye may get the embolus to move on. Call an eye doctor immediately to confirm the diagnosis and possibly tap the anterior chamber (paracentesis), which further lowers eye pressure. Refer the patient to an ER as soon as possible. It is not uncommon (27–76%) to also have a cerebral stroke.

Diabetic retinopathy

Fourteen percent of US adults have diabetes and another 40% have pre-diabetes. The high blood glucose levels may damage blood vessels throughout the body and can be best visualized in the retina. This disease can often be suspected in patients presenting with symptoms of insomnia, mood changes, frequent urination, thirst, slow healing and/or neuralgias. It may also be first detected on routine laboratory lab testing. One test called the HbA1C measures the 2–3 month average of glycosylated hemoglobin (Table 18, p.186) which could indicate diabetes if greater than 6.5% and pre- diabetes at levels of 5.7–6.4%. For each 1.0% increase in the HbA1C above those levels there is a 50% increase in complications A second confirmatory test is a fasting blood sugar (FBS) test taken after not eating for 8 Hrs. and it should be less than 120 mg/dl. Once diagnosed patients may also measure the FBS at home and the 2 hr postprandial (after meals) glucose which should be less than 180 mg/dl. The longer the sugar elevation is present the greater the risk of vessel toxicity. Up to 20% of patients may develop retinopathy after 10 years but since the exact date of onset of diabetes is not known the predictability of its course is mainly determined by keeping the HbA1C ideally less than 7.0%. With good control retinopathy doesn't have to occur even after 35 years. Control of body weight, cholesterol, and keeping blood pressure 10 mmHg lower than the normal standard at that age together with a regular exercise routine is also valuable. All diabetics should have a yearly dilated retina examination by an eye doctor.

Stage 1 Non-proliferative or background retinopathy is a microvascular breakdown of the blood-retina barrier, causing leakage of plasma and lipid with capillary dropout

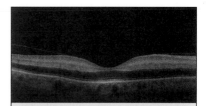

Fig 497 OCT of central retinal artery occlusion with inner retinal layer thickening due to cloudy swelling and a hyporeflective outer layer due to edema. *Source:* Courtesy of David Yarian, MD.

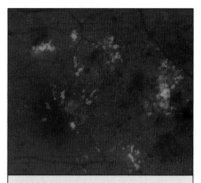

Fig 498 Stage 1: background retinopathy with microaneurysms, exudates, and dot hemorrhages. *Source:* Courtesy of Julia Monsonego, CRA, Wills Eye Hospital.

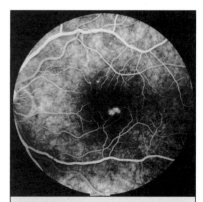

Fig 499 Leakage of fluorescein from microaneurysms. Normal retinal vessels do not leak.

(Figs 505 and 506). It initially presents with microaneurysms, dot hemorrhages, and exudates at the macula (see front cover image, Figs 498–501, and Fig. 536). These pale-yellow, hard lipid and protein leakages can be minimized by controlling serum lipids.

Macular edema (Fig. 500) is the most common cause of blindness before age 65 in the USA. Mild edema may first be treated with better control of blood sugar. If this is unsuccessful use intravitreal injections of anti-VEGF and less often corticosteroids Focal laser can be tried. The latter is reserved for cases where the edema is far enough away from the fovea as in Fig. 502 to prevent damage to this vital area of the retina. In cases unresponsive to any one treatment, a combination of these three may be given during a two-week period. Success is gauged by improved visual acuity and decreased thickness of the retina on OCT testing. Widespread capillary closure (Figs 505 and 506) causes ischemic infarcts of the nerve fiber layer resulting in cotton-wool spots, venous beading, blot hemorrhages, and the absence of blood flow on fluorescein angiography (Fig. 502).

Stage 2 Proliferative diabetic retinopathy (back cover) occurs when the ischemic areas of the retina stimulate the growth of abnormal curlicue capillaries on the surface of the retina (Figs 503, 560 and back cover), most often around the disk (back cover, Figs 502 and 503) and on the iris (Figs 388 and 389). The former may bleed into the vitreous and totally obstruct vision and the view of the retina. They then can cause fibrotic membranes (Figs 503 and 504) that contract, resulting in RDs. These new vessels are treated with panretinal photocoagulation (PRP) (back cover) that destroys part of the oxygen-demanding retina, thus reducing the release of VEGF that causes neovascularization. In PRP, 1500 laser burns are given in two sessions, often causing regression of neovascularization within several weeks. Intravitreal injection of anti-VEGF is an alternative treatment that also causes regression of new vessels. Laser is preferred in patients who may be non-compliant with the extended prolonged

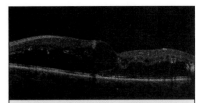

Fig 500 OCT of diffuse diabetic macular edema with hyporeflective (black) retinal thickening giving spongey appearance. *Source:* Courtesy of David Yarian, MD.

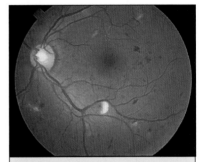

Fig 501 6 Stage 1: retinopathy with cotton-wool spots, microaneurysms, and dot hemorrhages.

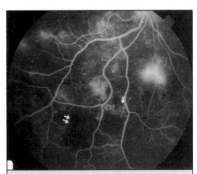

Fig 502 Fluorescein angiogram showing neovascularization (↓) adjacent to dark area of capillary nonperfusion (↓↓) and leakage of dye from vessels.

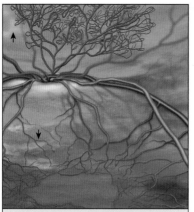

Fig 503 Stage 2: Proliferative retinopathy with preretinal neovascularization and pale ischemic areas (↑). Source: © 2021 JirehDesign. com. All Rights Reserved.

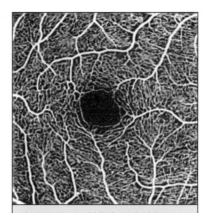

Fig 505 Normal black and white OCTA. Note ring of interconnected capillaries at the margin of the avascular fovea. *Source*: Courtesy of Carl Zeiss Meditec, Inc.

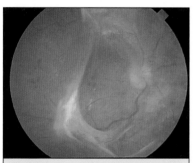

Fig 504 Stage 2: Bleeding into the vitreous may cause fibrous proliferation. These membranes may contract and cause RD.

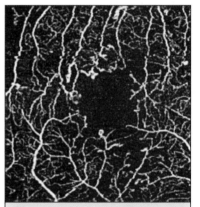

Fig 506 Black and white OCTA of diabetic retinopathy showing microaneurysms and area of ischemia appearing as darkened areas of nonperfusion. Also note widening of foveal avascular zone due to loss of capillaries. *Source*: Courtesy of Carl Zeiss Meditec, Inc.

number of visits needed with anti-VEGF injections. Stage 2 occurs late in the course of diabetes and is associated with other serious systemic vascular changes and an associated 56% 5-year survival rate. Diabetics should see an eye doctor annually for a retina examination through a dilated pupil.

To minimize these changes, one should be followed with careful control of blood sugar below 110 mg/dL, blood pressure less than 130/80 mmHg (10 mmHg less than non-diabetics), maintain normal cholesterol levels, exercise, stay thin, reduce abdominal obesity, and keep HbA1c levels ideally below 6.5% but less than

Table 18 Blood sugar levels in diabetes. 6.5% is diagnostic of diabetes but if glucose levels are kept below 7.0% it usually prevents vascular damage.	
Approximate equivalent	
HbA$_1$c (%)	*Mean non-fasting glucose (mg/dL)*
4	65
5	100
6	135
7	170
8	205
9.5	226
10.0	240
10.5	255
11.0	269
11.5	283

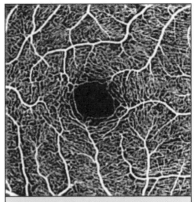

Fig 507 Normal black and white (OCT-A) of perifoveal retina. Normal black and white (OCT-A) of perifoveal retina. *Source*: Courtesy of Carl Zeiss Meditec, Inc.

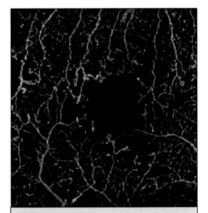

Fig 508 Diabetic retinopathy imaged with color OCTA showing microaneurysms and darkened ischemic areas of retinal capillary nonperfusion and enlargement of the foveal avascular zone, superficial retinal capillaries are red and deep retinal vessels are green. *Source*: Courtesy of Carl Zeiss Meditec, Inc.

7.0% often prevents problems. In an effort to get sugar levels too much below this value by increasing medication it sometimes results in sporadic hypoglycemia when glucose drops under 72mg/dl. This may result in dizziness, sweating, onfusion, increased heart rate, and even fainting and seizures. For each additional percentage point of HbA$_1$c, there is a 50% increase in complications. Lowering systolic BP by 10 mmHg, could reduce incidence of retinopathy by 40%.

Depth of retinal hemorrhages

Preretinal hemorrhages

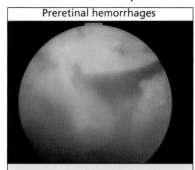

Fig 509 Pre-retinal hemorrhages lie between the retina internal limiting membrane and the posterior hyaloid surface of the vitreous. They may layer out to a boat shape. Common causes include a proliferative diabetic retinopathy, trauma, vitreous detachments, and leukemia (Fig. 528). This blood could break into the vitreous and obscure the view.

Superficial hemorrhages

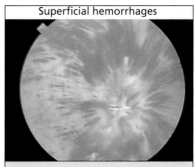

Fig 510 This central retinal vein occlusion shows superficial flame-shaped hemorrhages that follow the contour of the nerve fiber layer and radiate from the optic disk far out into the periphery. Flame hemorrhages also occur in papilledema, diabetes, hypertension, and optic neuritis, but do not extend to the peripheral retina as in central retinal vein occlusion.

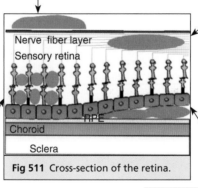

Nerve fiber layer
Sensory retina
RPE
Choroid
Sclera

Fig 511 Cross-section of the retina.

Deep retinal hemorrhages

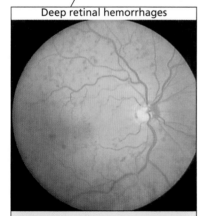

Fig 512 Intraretinal hemorrhages in partial central retinal vein occlusion.

Subretinal hemorrhages

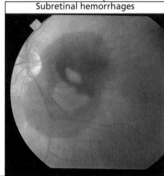

Fig 513 Wet macular degeneration with subretinal hemorrhages that are grayish in appearance since they are under the RPE. The red hemorrhages broke into the deep retina.

Age-related macular degeneration

Age-related macular degeneration (AMD) occurs after age 50 and is the leading cause of permanent blindness in elderly persons. Twenty-five percent of 70-year-old people have signs of the condition, and this number increases to 50% by age 90. It causes loss of central vision. In a normal retina (Fig. 514), the RPE has tight junctions protecting the sensory retina from leakage of more permeable choroidal capillaries. The RPE also metabolically supports the rods and cones, concentrates the vitamin A needed to regenerate the visual pigment rhodopsin and creates an adhesive force with the overlying neurosensory retina, which contains the rods and cones. This adhesion helps prevent RDs.

There are two types of AMD. The more common, the dry type, accounts for 90% of cases. In dry AMD, Bruch's membrane degenerates by fragmenting in some areas and thickening with hyaline (drusen) in other areas (Figs 515–517, 535, and 537). Drusen are deposits of waste products which increase with age. There is often pigment mottling and loss of the foveal reflex. The RPE on top of the drusen degenerates. Larger-sized drusen are considered more ominous. The overlying sensory retina, which is metabolically dependent on the RPE, thins out, resulting in atrophic macular degeneration. If enough retina disappears, the underlying choroidal vasculature is easily visualized with an ophthalmoscope. Advanced dry AMD is termed "geographic AMD" or "geographic atrophy" (Fig. 518) because of the large circumscribed atrophic areas through which choroidal vessels can be seen.

Dry AMD is treated with a combination of vitamin supplements sold OTC as a pill that includes Vit. A, which is naturally produced by plants, but not humans. It is the precursor of rhodopsin, the chemical in rods and cones, which when stimulated by light causes an electrical impulse responsible for a visual sensation. It also contains two other carotenoids,

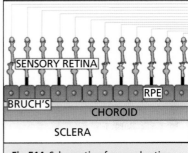

Fig 514 Schematic of normal retina showing retinal pigment epithelium sitting atop Bruch's membrane.

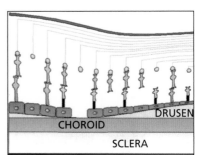

Fig 515 Dry AMD, with thinning of retina, thickening of Bruch's membrane (drusen) and disruption of RPE. The drusen are waste products of metabolism phagocytized by the RPE.

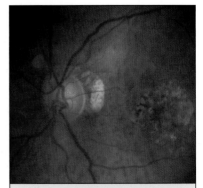

Fig 516 Dry AMD with pigment mottling, drusen, and loss of the foveal reflex. *Source*: Courtesy of Elliot Davidoff, MD.

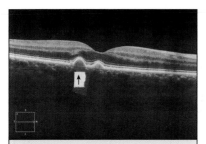

Fig 517 OCT of dry AMD with large drusen ↑. *Source*: Courtesy of Carl Zeiss, Meditec, Inc.

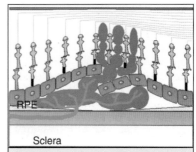

Fig 519 Neovascular (nAMD) is also called the *wet type*. Abnormal choroidal vessels elevate and then break through the RPE (Fig. 513).

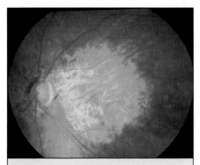

Fig 518 Geographic atrophy is the more advanced form of dry AMD resulting in atrophy of RPE with loss of overlying photoreceptors (rods and cones). The thinned RPE exposes underlying choroidal vasculature. *Source*: Courtesy of Elliot Davidoff, MD.

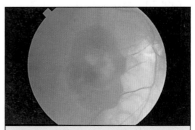

Fig 520 Hemorrhagic stage of wet AMD may be associated with severe vision loss and fibrous scarring (Fig. 525).

zeaxanthin and lutein, which support the rods and cones. Vitamins E and C serve as antioxidants and the zinc additive may help neuronal development. This combination pill has been shown to reduce visual loss by 25%. Dry AMD progression also benefits from minimizing exposure to UV light and cessation of cigarette smoking.

About 10% of the early dry AMD may progress to geographic atrophy and/or to the wet type, also referred to as *neovascular AMD* (nAMD), in which abnormal choroidal blood vessels (subretinal neovascularization) form (Figs 519–524). The goal is to recognize these vessels before they bleed and cause a hemorrhagic detachment of the RPE, which appear dark grayish-red (Fig. 513). When they penetrate the RPE into the sensory retina, they

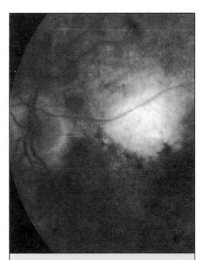

Fig 521 Fluorescein angiogram of subretinal neovascular membrane.

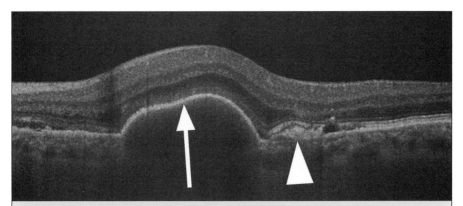

Fig 522 OCT of wet AMD with increased retinal thickening due to edema (appears black); pigment epithelial detachment (↑) with significant elevation; penetration of pigment epithelial layer by choroidal vessels (∧). *Source*: Courtesy of David Yarian, MD.

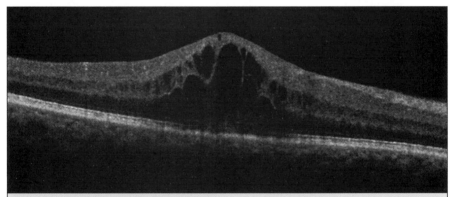

Fig 523 OCT of wet AMD with cystoid macular edema. This loculated type of edema also occurs in diabetes, retinal vein occlusions, uveitis, and most commonly in 2–60% of cataract surgeries during the immediate post-operative period. Steroids and non-steroidal anti-inflammatories routinely given after cataract surgery resolve almost all post-op macular edema.

appear bright red (Fig. 520). Eventually, the blood could fibrose and form a white scar (Fig. 525) called *disciform macular degeneration*, resulting in permanent loss of vision. An early symptom of progression from the dry to wet form may be that straight lines become wavy on the Amsler grid which can be given to patients for home testing (see Figs 131 and 590).

The initial treatment for wet AMD is a monthly or less frequent intravitreal injection of an anti-VEGF (Figs 526 and 527) for an as-yet-undetermined—perhaps indefinite—number

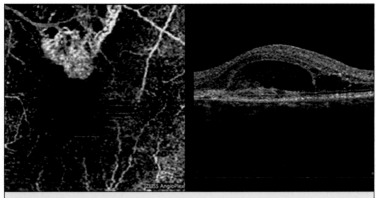

Fig 524 AMD imaged with OCTA showing choroidal neovascularization on left and elevation of RPE on right. This may also occur in pathologic myopia and presumed histoplasmosis. *Source:* Courtesy of Carl Zeiss, Meditec. Inc.

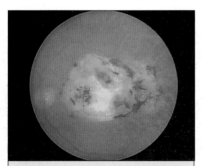

Fig 525 Late-stage wet AMD with disciform scar following hemorrhage.

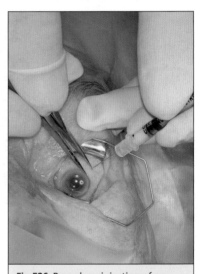

Fig 526 Pars plana injection of an anti-VEGF to treat wet AMD. Calipers measure a site 3.5 mm posterior to the limbus in the space between the retina and vascular ciliary body. *Source:* Courtesy of Elliot Davidoff, MD.

of months. Patients have already been reported to have had 109 injections. This drug antagonizes VEGF, causing regression of abnormal vessels. The time between injections may be increased (treat-and-extend) depending on findings at follow-up visits. It prevents progression of angiogenesis in most cases, but only 30–40% of patients get improvement in vision.

If anti-VEGF therapy is not effective, laser photodynamic therapy may be used. Intravenously administered verteporfin (Visudyne) concentrates in the new vessels. A low-energy laser is then aimed at the vessels, activating the dye, causing most cell death inside the vessel, but also some collateral retinal damage. Laser is usually reserved for non-central edema that is far enough away from the fovea to minimize

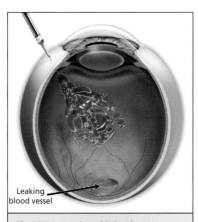

Leaking
blood vessel

Fig 527 Intravitreal injections are becoming the most common intraocular ophthalmic procedure performed in the USA, doubling that of cataract surgery. Besides anti-VEGF, which is the most common medication injected into the vitreous, others include the steroids (triamcinolone and dexamethasone) (Fig. 367); the antivirals (ganciclovir and foscarnet), used to treat herpes and cytomegalovirus; the antibiotics (vancomycin, ceftazidime, and amikacin); and the antifungal (amphotericin B). These injections may cause serious infections (endophthalmitis), pressure elevation, retinal detachment, and traumatic cataract.

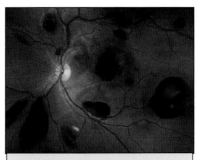

Fig 528 White-centered pre-retinal hemorrhages called *Roth spots* may occur in anemia, leukemia, diabetes, hypertension, and bacterial endocarditis, in which case septic emboli damage the vessel wall. The pale center is due to fibrin. *Source*: Courtesy of Debra Brown, COT, CRA, University of San Francisco.

loss of central vision. Besides wet AMD, Visudyne/ laser therapy is used to treat choroidal neovascularization in pathologic myopia and presumed histoplasmosis (Figs 409 and 524).

Rarer causes of macular degeneration are juvenile inherited types, such as Stargardt's disease (the most common); chorioretinitis; infection; and staring at the sun. Reassure patients that they never go totally blind from macular disease, but only lose the central field, often resulting in 20/400 vision.

Central serous chorioretinopathy

Central serous chorioretinopathy (Figs 529–532) is a relatively common macular disease in which a defect in the RPE allows choroidal fluid to leak into the sensory retina. The incidence is six times higher in men, often aged 25–40, and may be triggered by corticosteroids and stress. Symptoms are decreased and distorted vision. Wavy lines are demonstrated with an Amsler grid (Figs 131 and 590). Ophthalmoscopically, it is difficult to visualize the clear, oval elevation of the retina. It is easily diagnosed with fluorescein angiography (Fig. 530) or the less invasive OCT (Fig. 532). Eighty to ninety percent clear within 3 months. Photodynamic laser therapy may be used if leakage continues for 6 months. It may recur and become chronic about 40% of the time.

Pseudoxanthoma elasticum

Pseudoxanthoma elasticum is a systemic disease. There may be cardiovascular abnormalities, gastrointestinal hemorrhages, and loose skin folds on the neck (Fig. 539). The retina may have angioid streaks (Fig. 538), which also occur in Ehlers–Danlos, Paget's, and sickle cell disease.

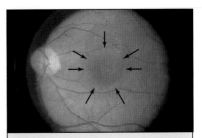

Fig 529 Central serous chorioretinopathy.

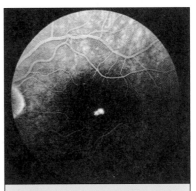

Fig 530 Fluorescein leakage through the RPE in central serous chorioretinopathy, often appearing as a single "smoke stack."

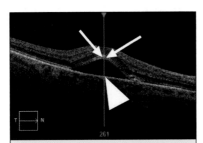

Fig 532 OCT of central serous chorioretinopathy showing subretinal fluid detaching the sensory retina epithelium (↑↑) and thickening of the choriocapillaries with thinning of the RPE (∧). This thickening of the choroidal layer is due to large dysfunctional vessels and it is referred to as *pachychoroid* (*pachy* is Greek for thick, as used in describing an elephant's skin—pachyderm). This anatomical disorder, recently described in 2020, is also associated with other less common retinal diseases. *Source*: Courtesy of David Yarian, MD.

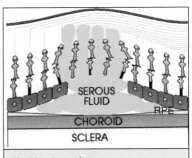

Fig 531 Central serous chorioretinopathy.

White and yellow retinal lesions

Cotton-wool spots

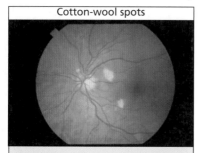

Fig 533 Cotton-wool spots in AIDS. Arteriolar closure causes infarctions of the superficial nerve fiber layer. These white, cloud-like lesions cluster around the disk and obscure the underlying retina (see Figs 4, 482, 486, and cover).

Inflammatory cells

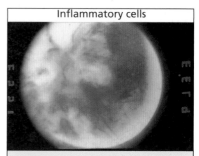

Fig 534 White, inflammatory cells in cytomegalovirus retinitis. *Source*: Courtesy of Joseph Walsh, MD.

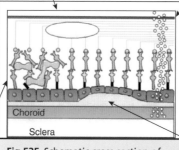

Choroid

Sclera

Fig 535 Schematic cross-section of retina.

Hard (waxy) exudate

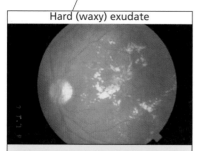

Fig 536 Exudate in background diabetic retinopathy. Leaking fluid from vessels leaves behind an irregularly shaped, waxy, yellowish lipoprotein residue. It is seen most often in diabetes and retinal vein occlusions (See front cover).

Retinal drusen

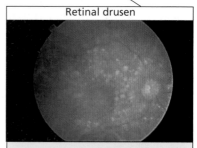

Fig 537 Drusen, together with pigment mottling and decreased vision is often a first warning of macular degeneration. Drusen are small, white, round, often bilateral and uniformly distributed. They must be distinguished from waxy exudates that are yellow, irregular in shape, and distribution is also frequently in the macula.

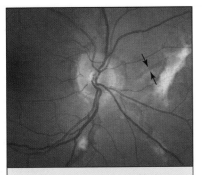

Fig 538 Pseudoxanthoma elasticum: Angloid streaks are breaks in Bruch's membrane (↑) that radiate from the peripapillary area. This disease can cause retinopathy and loss of vision. *Source*: Courtesy of Julia Monsonego, CRA, Wills Eye Hospital.

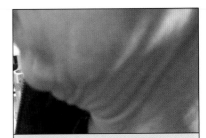

Fig 539 Do not confuse pseudoxanthoma elasticum and Ehlers–Danlos (ED) syndrome. Both are inherited diseases of the skin elasticity (loose skin on the neck), arterial aneurysms, blue sclera, and retinal angioid streaks. Unique to Ehlers–Danlos is hyperextensibility of the joints.

Albinism

Albinism has many forms and refers to inherited hypopigmentation. Common findings in all types involving the eye are photophobia, hypopigmentation of the retina (Fig. 540), and transillumination of the iris with a penlight at the limbus (Fig. 541). Additional findings may include nystagmus, a hypoplastic macula with the absence of a foveal reflex, reduced vision, refractive errors, decreased immunity, and decreased pigmentation of the hair and skin (Fig. 542).

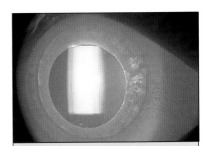

Fig 541 Transilluminated iris in albinism.

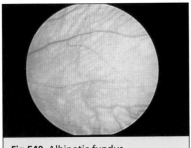

Fig 540 Albinotic fundus.

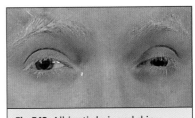

Fig 542 Albinotic hair and skin.

Retinitis pigmentosa

Retinitis pigmentosa (Figs 543–546) is a slowly progressive hereditary rod and cone degeneration. Inheritance patterns include autosomal dominant or recessive and X-linked recessive. Since it begins in the retinal periphery, the first loss is peripheral and night vision, often sparing central visual acuity for many years. The retina has pigmentary changes resembling bone corpuscles. The diagnosis is confirmed with an electroretinogram. Treatment with supplements and medications is as yet not proven to be effective.

Researchers have restored some vision in blind humans with implantation of silicon microchips in the subretinal or epiretinal space to convert light energy into electrical current (Fig. 546). The Argus II epiretinal prosthesis was recently approved by the US Food and Drug Administration. By 2019, four hundred have been implanted. Patients often have regained the ability to see shapes of a cup, walk without help, and have improved social interactions.

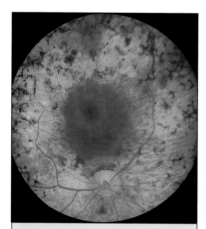

Fig 543 Retinitis pigmentosa with bony pigmented spicules. *Source:* Courtesy of John Fingert, MD, and *Arch. Ophthalmol.*, Sept. 2008, Vol. 126, No. 9, pp. 1301–1303.

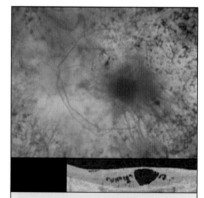

Fig 544 Retinitis pigmentosa with macular cyst clearly visible on OCT. *Source:* Courtesy of Alexis Smith, CRA, OCT-C, Kellogg Eye Center, Ann Arbor, MI.

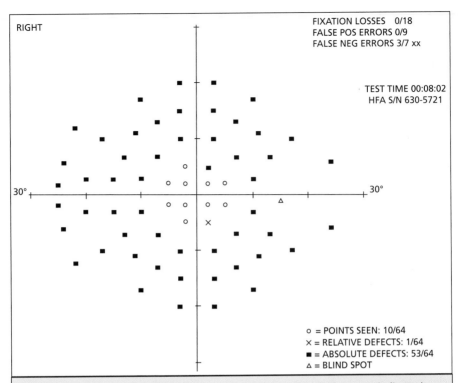

FIXATION LOSSES   0/18
FALSE POS ERRORS 0/9
FALSE NEG ERRORS 3/7 xx

TEST TIME 00:08:02
HFA S/N 630-5721

RIGHT

30°

30°

○ = POINTS SEEN: 10/64
✕ = RELATIVE DEFECTS: 1/64
■ = ABSOLUTE DEFECTS: 53/64
△ = BLIND SPOT

Fig 545 Constricted visual field in late-stage retinitis pigmentosa. Dark squares indicate the absence of vision.

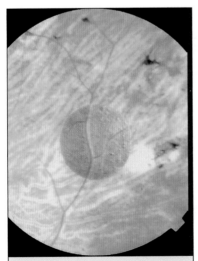

Fig 546 A microchip in the subretinal space (note black pigment clumping typical of retinitis pigmentosa). *Source*: Courtesy of Alan and Vincent Chow.

Retinoblastoma

This is a malignant tumor of the retina, often appearing by 2 years of age. Most arise from a genetic mutation that survivors may transmit in a Mendelian dominant fashion. There may be one or more white, elevated retinal masses which are bilateral 30% of the time (Fig. 547). A CT scan often reveals calcifications in the tumor. In the past, enucleation (Figs 423–426) was a primary treatment. Now attempts at salvaging some vision and the globe are replacing enucleation with injection of chemotherapeutic agents into the ophthalmic artery, radiation therapy, laser therapy, cryotherapy, and intravitreal chemo-injections. All infants at 3 and 6 months should be tested for a red pupillary reflex, which should reveal symmetric red reflections with no opacities (Fig. 548). Family members should get genetic counseling.

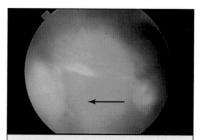

Fig 547 Retinoblastoma. *Source:* Courtesy of David Taylor.

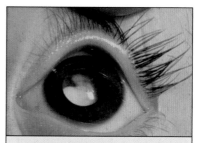

Fig 548 Leukocoria (white pupil) due to retinoblastoma.

Retinopathy of prematurity

Retinopathy of prematurity (ROP) is a disease of newborns that occurs in premature infants weighing less than 1500 g or having a gestational age of 28 weeks or less. It occurs more often when oxygen is administered.

Normal vascularization of the retina progresses peripherally and is not normally completed until 1 month after birth. Oxygen given to newborns stops this normal vascularization process. When the oxygen is discontinued, the avascular peripheral retina stimulates new vessel growth (Figs 549 and 550). These new vessels, however, are now abnormal and may bleed, resulting in vitreous hemorrhage with fibrous proliferation. It can drag the retina (Fig. 551), sometimes causing a RD. The ideal therapy is comprehensive prenatal care to reduce the number of premature births and careful monitoring of oxygen in the nursery.

ROP is becoming more prevalent because of advances in neonatal intensive care, which have led to an improvement in survival for

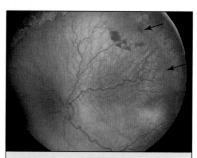

Fig 549 Stage 3 retinopathy of prematurity (ROP). Note line of demarcation where normal retinal vessels stopped growing (↑). It is initially a flat line (stage 1), then it forms a ridge (stage 2) before abnormal vessels start growing (stage 3). Laser treatment will hopefully prevent a stage 4 retinal detachment. Stage 5 is total retinal detachment.

very low birthweight infants. An eye doctor should check the peripheral retina at 6 weeks of a baby's chronological age or 32 weeks gestational age, whichever was earlier.

Laser photocoagulation of the peripheral retina is presently the first-line treatment of the avascular retina in stage 3 when the demarcation line is elevated with fibrovascular proliferation (Fig. 551). Increasingly, anti-VEGF injections into the vitreous are being evaluated. Rigid examination and treatment guidelines and frequent poor visual outcomes are causing a shortage of doctors willing to follow these infants and be exposed to high-cost litigation. A web-based telemedicine system is presently being evaluated. Retinal photographs taken by nurses and technicians are being sent to remote sites to be reviewed by experts.

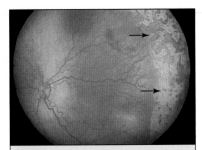

Fig 550 Regression of abnormal vessels and hemorrhages after treating ischemic peripheral retina with laser (↑). *Source*: Courtesy of Anna L. Ellis, MD, and *Arch. Ophthalmol.*, Oct. 2002, Vol. 120, p. 1405. Copyright 2002, American Medical Association.

Vitreous

The vitreous is a clear gel that is 98% water. The viscosity is due to hyaluronic acid and collagen fibrils. It fills the interior of the globe like air fills a balloon. The vitreous normally liquefies and shrinks in 63% of people over age 70 causing floaters and flashing lights due to traction of the retina (Fig. 552). The floaters commonly result in a visual sensation of shifting particles that are annoying, but rarely severe enough to require treatment. Removal of the vitreous with a surgical pars plana vitrectomy (Figs 553–555) is rarely performed for these symptoms because of significant side effects requiring a return to the operating room for cataract surgery in 3.7% of cases and retinal detachment 2.6%.of the time.

The pars plana vitrectomy is performed in the operating room. Three instruments are inserted into the eye through the anterior pars plana. This location avoids the highly vascular ciliary processes, and the delicate retina. The entry sites are located on the sclera by measuring 3.5 mm posterior to the limbus. One instrument is for endoillumination. The second is for irrigation with balance saline to replace any vitreous removed. The third portal allows for instruments that cut and remove

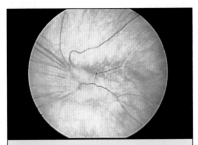

Fig 551 Late stage retinopathy of prematurity with disk and retinal vessels dragged peripherally.

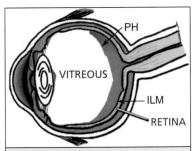

Fig 552 Posterior vitreous detachment. The posterior surface of the vitreous is called the *posterior hyaloid* (PH) and is made up of condensed collagen fibers. The membrane covering the adjacent retinal surface is called the *internal limiting membrane* (ILM).

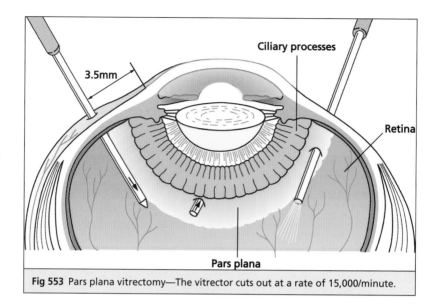

Fig 553 Pars plana vitrectomy—The vitrector cuts out at a rate of 15,000/minute.

Fig 554 Pars plana vitrectomy showing sites for illumination, irrigation, and aspiration. The interior of the eye is viewed using a cornea contact lens together with the operating microscope. *Source:* Courtesy of Stuart Green, MD.

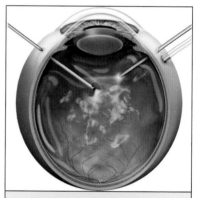

Fig 555 Pars plana vitrectomy. *Source:* JirehDesign.com.

vitreous membranes; obtain tissue for cytology or culture; inject medications, gas or silicone oil; cauterize or laser photocoagulate the retina; and forceps and/or magnets to remove foreign bodies.

A newer, safer method to treat floaters is called *laser vitreolysis* (Figs 556 and 557). However, it is only reserved for persistent (4–5 months), often solitary, floaters in the visual axis that aren't too close to the retina or back surface of the lens and are causing significant symptoms. It has limited success since it does not remove floaters, but only renders them smaller.

Patients with floaters and flashes present on an almost daily basis (Fig. 556). They require a dilated retina exam since about 1 in 20 may have pathology requiring treatment. Infrequently, floaters could be due to inflammation from choroiditis (Fig. 559); retinitis or vitreous hemorrhage (Figs 560 and 561), asteroid hyalosis, trauma, and a retinal hole or detachment.

In asteroid hyalosis, hundreds of small, spherical balls are suspended in the vitreous and, amazingly, aren't very annoying to the patient. When questioned, they admit to seeing floaters (Fig. 558). These calcium phospholipid crystals deposit in the vitreous for no apparent reason and are benign. They appear like stars in the galaxy with an ophthalmoscope or slit lamp and requires no treatment.

Inflammatory cell in vitreous due to choroiditis and retinitis may obscure the view of the retina. Hemorrhages, most often due to diabetes, and retinal tears also restrict the view. B-scan ultrasound can be useful for eyes with vitreous haze (Fig. 560).

The vitreous is most strongly adherent to the retina at the vitreous base (near the ora serrata), and less so at the macula, and the optic disk. A posterior vitreous detachment (PVD) occurs in 63% of people and could tear

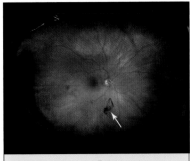

Fig 556 Vitreous opacity.

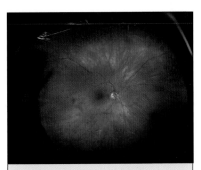

Fig 557 Vitreolysis of vitreous opacity with laser breaking it up into smaller particles *Source*: Courtesy of Chirag Shah, MD.

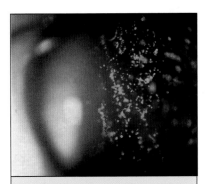

Fig 558 Slit lamp view of asteroid hyalosis with lens seen on left and vitreous on right.

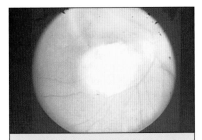

Fig 559 Hazy view of toxoplasmosis choroiditis due to white cells in the vitreous.

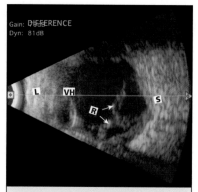

Fig 560 Vitreous hemorrhage or inflammatory cells could hinder one from getting a clear view of the retina. B-scan ultrasound of retinal detachment (R) with vitreous hemorrhage (VH), posterior surface of lens (L), and sclera (S).

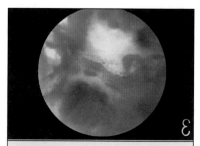

Fig 561 Blunt trauma, causing pre-, intra-, and subretinal hemorrhages is referred to as a *commotio retinae*. Hemorrhage may extend into the vitreous. Traumatic hemorrhages also occur in 85% of cases of abusive head trauma, previously referred to as *shaken-baby syndrome*, and must be looked for when physical abuse is suspected (Table 6, p. 53).

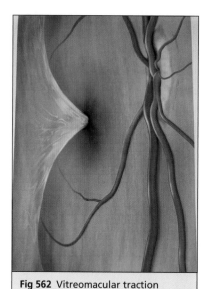

Fig 562 Vitreomacular traction

the very thin superficial internal limiting membrane (ILM) covering the retina at these locations (Fig. 552). Breaks to the ILM allow glial cells to grow onto the surface of the retina. These epiretinal membranes (ERMs) occur in 34% of adults over 63 years of age. This gliosis at first is a clear, glistening, cellophane-like membrane that can then progress to

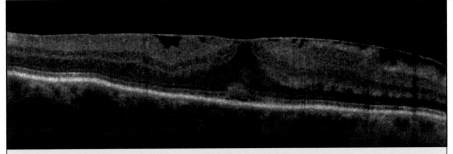

Fig 563 OCT of epiretinal membrane appearing as a thickened white line on surface of the retina. Contraction causing pucker due to wrinkling and thickening of retina from macular edema. A macular hole could result. Source: Courtesy of David Yarian, MD

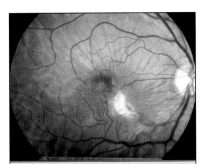

Fig 564 Macular pucker with visible traction lines It occurs in 6% of the population.

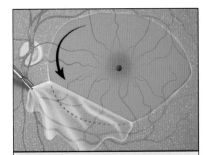

Fig 566 A circular tear then peels off the opacified epithelial membrane with or without the ILM. Illustration by Chris Gralapp.

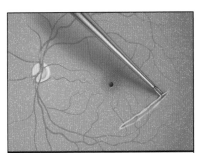

Fig 565 A blade or forceps is used to create an initial flap in the internal limiting membrane. Triamcinolone crystals or FDA-approved TissueBlue dye may be injected to coat the membrane for easier identification. Illustration by Chris Gralapp.

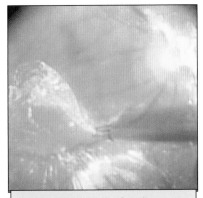

Fig 567 Photograph of peeling epiretinal membrane. *Source:* M.E. Parah, M. Maia, and E.B. Rodrigues, *Am. J. Ophthalmol,* 2009, Vol. 148, No. 3, p. 338. Reproduced with permission of Elsevier.

a more translucent, and then opaque, membrane (Figs 564–567) that can reduce vision. The ERM can contract and cause macular pucker with wrinkling of the retina (Figs 562–564), distortion of vision, and a macular hole (Figs 562, 568, 569, and 570). If vision is significantly affected, surgical vitrectomy and membranectomy can be performed (Figs 565–567).

Retinal holes

Retinal holes (Figs 571 and 572) are treated differently depending on the size and location. Fluid often enters the hole (Fig. 573) and could cause a RD. Small, asymptomatic peripheral holes, with no RD, may be observed with no treatment. Larger peripheral holes may be treated with a laser or transconjunctival cryotherapy to surround holes with a barrier of chorioretinal scars (Figs 576 and 577). This scarring treatment cannot be used for macular holes since it would damage central vision.

Vitreous or epiretinal membrane traction could cause a macular hole (Figs 562, 568 and 569). These can resolve on its own by the spontaneous lysis of vitreous adhesion or it can lead to macular cysts and partial- or full-thickness holes. Partial-thickness holes (lamellar holes) in the macula can partially reduce vision and may be observed without treatment (Fig. 572). However, 70% may progress to full thickness with severe loss of central vision. A vitrectomy (Figs 553-555 and 579) with the removal of any epiretinal membrane, with or without the internal limiting membrane (Figs. 564–567) may be performed to release traction. A gas is then injected into the vitreous and the patient is sent home to lie on their stomach for 2 weeks so that the air rises and tamponades the hole preventing intraocular fluid from entering. This in turn allows for absorption of fluid so that the edges of the hole can fuse. Ninety percent of holes close, achieving visual acuity of 20/50 or better and may keep improving for up to three years after surgery. A newer, non-surgical alternative in symptomatic cases is to lyse

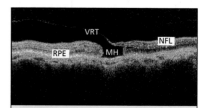

Fig 568 OCT scan of full-thickness macular hole with no detachment caused by vitreous traction. RPE (retinal pigment epithelium; NFL (nerve fiber layer); MH (macular hole); VRT (vitreoretinal traction).

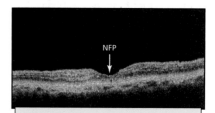

Fig 569 OCT scan of macular hole resolution after vitrectomy with injection of gas into the vitreous. NFP (normal foveal pit).

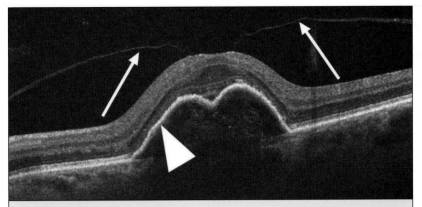

Fig 570 OCT showing vitreomacular traction (↑) with pigment epithelial detachment (A) and fluid. There is macular edema causing loss of foveal pit, but no hole yet. *Source*: Courtesy of David Yarian, MD.

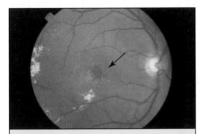

Fig 571 Diabetic retinopathy with exudates and macular hole (↑).

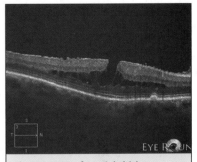

Fig 572 OCT of partial-thickness macular hole, called a *lamellar hole*. Also, note white epiretinal membrane on the surface of retina creating traction. *Source*: Courtesy of University of Iowa, Eyerounds.org.

vitreomacular adhesions by injection of a proteolytic enzyme (ocriplasmin – Jetrea) into the vitreous. Cost and side effects have limited widespread acceptance.

In 12% of cases of posterior vitreous detachment, the tear is more severe than just the ILM and extends partway (Figs 562 and 572) through the sensory retina. Of these partial retinal holes, 70% go on to develop into full-thickness holes (Fig. 568).

The liberation of orange pigment from the RPE may be seen in the vitreous at the slit lamp as clumps of tobacco-like dust. It indicates a greater possibility of a full-thickness hole mandating a most thorough examination to find the source of the pigment. Similarly, if white or red cells are seen, a site of origin should be sought.

Retinal detachment

Symptoms of RD often include loss of vision, described as a "curtain", with flashes and floaters. Ophthalmoscopically, it appears as an elevated, gray membrane, unless a vitreous hemorrhage obscures it.

A RD is a separation of the neurosensory retina containing the rods and cones from the underlying RPE (Figs 462, 485, 573-578). There is normally a low-grade adhesion between these two layers, which can be broken by traction allowing fluid to enter the space between them. Sixty-six percent of RDs begin with myopic thinning of lattice degeneration in the peripheral retina. Lattice degeneration is seen with an indirect ophthalmoscope in 8% of eyes as a white meshwork of lines with black pigment near the ora serrata (Fig. 574). Holes may develop in these areas spontaneously or from trauma, cataract surgery, vitreous traction, or contraction of diabetic retinal membranes (Fig. 504). Fluid enters the holes and detaches the retina. This

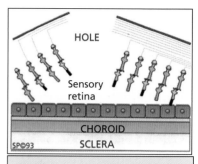

Fig 573 Retinal hole with detachment of sensory retina from pigment epithelium.

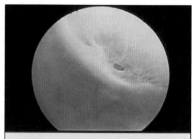

Fig 574 Lattice degeneration, with a small, round hole with fluid entering the hole and detaching the retina. *Source*: Courtesy of Leo Bores

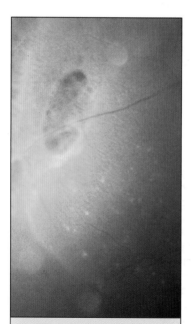

Fig 575 Retinal detachment caused by a large tear and hole in area of lattice degeneration.

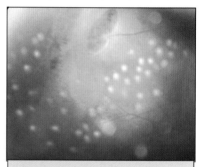

Fig 576 Pneumatic retinopathy is performed in office. After laser photocoagulation or cryotherapy barrier treatment of the hole, the retinal detachment in the previous figure is treated with air or the expansile gas C³F and positioning of the body so that the bubble rises and tamponades the tear. *Source*: Courtesy of Jiuhn-Feng Hwang, MD and San-Ni Chen, MD. Reprinted from *Am. J. Ophthalmol.*, Feb. 2007, Vol. 143, No. 2, pp. 117–221.

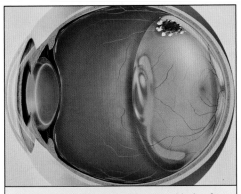

Fig 577 Bubble tamponading retinal hole after laser treatment creates barrier scar around hole.

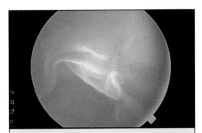

Fig 578 Retinal detachment with a large hole referred to as horseshoe tear. A must to be treated as opposed to small, round, holes that are asymptomatic and probably old.

is called *rhegmatogenous RD* (*rhegm* is Greek for broken).

Fifteen percent of all small RDs (Fig. 576), especially with small holes and no vitreous traction, can be repaired with pneumatic retinopexy. A gas is injected into the vitreous as an office procedure (Fig. 577). It presses the retina against the choroid and tamponades the hole by manipulating the patient's head position. The air prevents fluid from entering the hole and is absorbed in several days. In office laser is used to seal the hole with a chorioretinal barrier scar that surrounds the hole (Figs 576 and 577). If there is vitreous traction a vitrectomy (Figs 553–555, and 579) may be performed.

Very large RDs with multiple and/or giant tears (Fig. 578) are treated by adopting a more complicated procedure called *scleral buckle* (Fig. 580). In this procedure, a scleral flap is created through which subretinal fluid is drained. This allows for immediate apposition of the retina to pigment epithelium. Transscleral cryotherapy creates a barrier scar around the hole and a buckle is placed around the globe to indent the sclera against the retina (Fig. 581). A vitrectomy with a bubble of air is often injected to manipulate the retina and is absorbed in several days. The expansive gas, C^3F, when needed lasts for

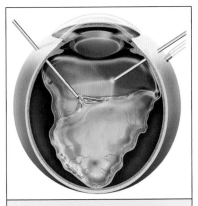

Fig 579 Retinal detachment due to contraction of vitreous membranes treated with pars plana vitrectomy. *Source*: Jireh Design.com.

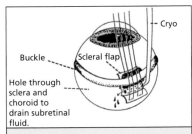

Cryo

Buckle

Scleral flap

Hole through sclera and choroid to drain subretinal fluid.

Fig 580 Scleral buckling repair of retinal detachment.

weeks. Silicone oil is also used for tissue manipulation in the most complicated cases. It must be removed in 2–3 months, once the retinal anatomy is stable since it could migrate to the anterior chamber causing glaucoma, keratitis, and adherence of oil droplets to an intraocular lens.

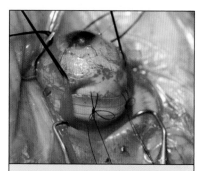

Fig 581 Repair of retinal detachment with silicone buckle. *Source:* Courtesy of Stuart Green, MD

Appendix 1
Hyperlipidemia

Normal blood lipids

Normal cholesterol	<199 mg/dL
HDL cholesterol	>39 mg/dL
LDL cholesterol	<99 mg/dL
LDL/HDL ratio	<3.6
Triglycerides	<150 mg/dL

The two carotid arteries are the main blood supply to the brain and the most common site liberating emboli that cause ischemic stroke. A carotid endarterectomy may be performed to remove atherosclerotic plaque buildup from one or both carotid arteries.

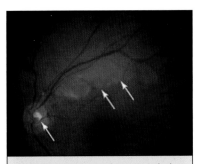

Fig 582 Branch retinal artery embolus (↑) from carotid artery and resulting pale ischemic retina (↑↑). *Source*: Courtesy of Elliot Davidoff, MD.

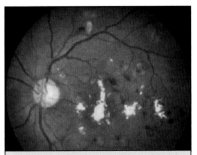

Fig 583 In diabetes, hard exudates are caused by lipoproteins leaking from retinal capillaries into the extracellular space. Lowering blood fat levels helps minimize this complication. *Source*: Courtesy of Joanna Gostyla.

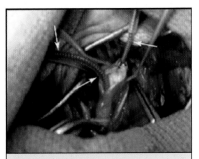

Fig 584 Carotid endarterectomy showing temporary shunt (↑) to bypass surgical site. It is the gold standard for treating carotid stenosis. If contraindicated, stenting is considered. *Source*: Courtesy of Niranjan Rao, MD, St. Peter's University Hospital.

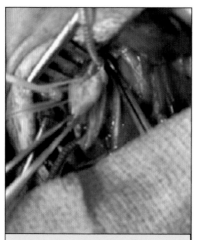

Fig 585 Thrombectomy using spatula and forceps (see Fig. 135).

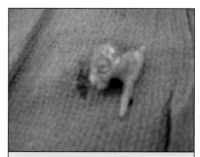

Fig 586 Plaque removed from carotid artery.

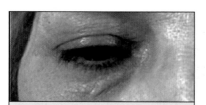

Fig 587 Xanthelasma are irregular yellowish plaque on the medial side of the upper and lower lids. They are often inherited and sometimes associated with hypercholesterolemia and a 51% increased risk of heart attack.

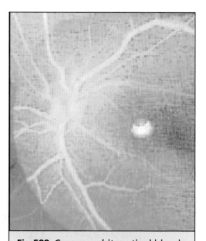

Fig 588 Creamy, white retinal blood vessels indicating lipemia retinalis which occurs with triglyceride levels >2500 mg/dL. This patient had triglycerides of 29,000 mg/dL and cholesterol of 1470 mg/dL. *Source*: Courtesy of Murat Ozdemir, MD, and *Ophthalmic Surg. Lasers Imaging*, 2003, Vol. 34, pp. 221–222.

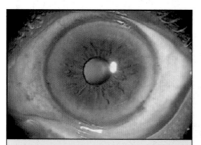

Fig 589 Corneal arcus is a narrow, white band of lipid infiltration separated from the limbus by a clear zone. It occurs in everyone by age 80. Its occurrence in those younger than 50 warrants measuring blood lipids, which may be elevated.

Appendix 2
Amsler grid

1 Wear best corrected lenses for near vision.
2 Hold card at 35 cm.
3 Cover one eye.
4 Focus on central dot.
5 Detect any wavy, distorted, or blind areas.

Wavy lines and loss of vision often indicate a progression of dry to wet macular degeneration. Lines may also become curved in other macular diseases and cataracts which are often present in this same age group.

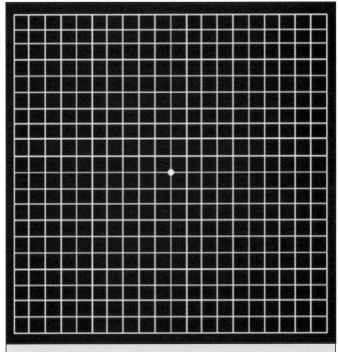

Fig 590 Amsler grid.

Manual for Eye Examination and Diagnosis, Tenth Edition. Mark W. Leitman.
© 2021 John Wiley & Sons Ltd. Published 2021 by John Wiley & Sons Ltd.

Index

Page numbers in *italics* refer to figures. Search by page or figure number.